AF566940

NEUROBLASTOMA RESEARCH TRENDS

NEUROBLASTOMA RESEARCH TRENDS

LUCAS H. ANDRE
AND
NATHAN E. ROUX
EDITORS

Nova Biomedical Books
New York

For permission to use material from this book please contact us:
Telephone 631-231-7269; Fax 631-231-8175
Web Site: http://www.novapublishers.com

Library of Congress Cataloging-in-Publication Data

Neuroblastoma research trends / [edited by] Lucas H. Andre and Nathan E. Roux. p. ; cm.
Includes bibliographical references and index.
ISBN 978-1-60456-790-8 (hardcover)
1. Neuroblastoma. 2. Cancer cells. I. Andre, Lucas H. II. Roux, Nathan E.
[DNLM: 1. Neuroblastoma. QZ 380 N4932 2008]
RC280.N4N4847 2008
616.99'48--dc22 *2008025938*

Published by Nova Science Publishers, Inc., New York

Contents

Preface

Neuroblastoma is a cancer that develops from nerve cells found in several areas of the body. Neuroblastoma most commonly affects children age 5 or younger, though it may rarely occur in older children and adults. Neuroblastoma is the most common cancer in babies. Neuroblastoma develops in tissue that makes up the sympathetic nervous system — the system of nerves that automatically regulates your heart rate, blood pressure and digestion. Neuroblastoma most commonly arises in and around the adrenal glands, which sit atop the kidneys. However, neuroblastoma can also develop in other areas of the abdomen and in the chest, neck and pelvis. This new book presents important new research in this field of research.

Chapter I - Neuroblastoma (NB) is a common pediatric solid tumor. Macroscopically as well as microscopically, NB shows a heterogeneous appearance. One important question is what the basis of this heterogeneity is. Another question is how this heterogeneity influences the biological characteristics and/or treatment strategy for NB. Recently, the first question has been well answered by the cancer stem cell theory. That is to say that cancer originates from a stem cell with the ability of self-renewal as well as multipotency. The cancer comprises a hierarchical organization with only a small number of cancer stem cells (CSCs) and a large number of their descendants. Only the CSCs are responsible for tumorigenicity, progression and metastasis in the cancer, while their descendants are not. Their descendants will differentiate, resulting in the heterogeneity of the cancer. Recently, CSCs have been isolated from some cancers. The real target determining the biological characteristics and the treatment strategy should be the CSCs themselves instead of the rest (and the majority) of the constituent cancer cells. Normal stem cells and CSCs show similar resistance to current therapies, because they both stay in a quiescent state and have a common drug efflux capacity. This means that a small fraction of cancer stem cells can survive aggressive therapies, even though the remaining majority of the cancer cells are responsive to them. This eventually leads to relapse of the cancer. If this is the case with NB, isolation of the CSCs in NB is the first step for understanding their characteristics and for developing treatment strategies for them. Side population (SP) cells characterized by the efficient efflux of Hoechst 33342 dye are thought to be enriched for stem cells in many normal tissues. Recently, SP cells that showed stem cell characteristics were isolated from primary NB tumors as well as NB cell lines. The authors have also investigated SP cells in NB cell lines and found that NB cell lines contained a small fraction of SP cells. Furthermore, normal stem cells as well as CSCs are believed to be maintained by the microenvironment surrounding them (called the "niche"). It will be now important to focus on not only the small fraction of CSCs but also their niche in NB in order to characterize their biological behavior and to developing strategies to eradicate the tumor. A new era in neuroblastoma research has begun with the establishment of the cancer stem cell theory. The diagnostic and therapeutic implications of CSCs in NB are herein reviewed and discussed.

Chapter II - Neuroblastoma, the third most common paediatric solid tumors after leukaemiae and brain neoplasiae, with an incidence of approximately 1.3 child out of 100.000, is responsible of 15% of all childhood cancer death.

The acquisition of multidrug resistance upon treatment with anticancer drugs is a common feature of highly malignant Neuroblastoma. The identification of marker proteins involved in chemo-resistance might significantly help in the prognosis of this neoplasia by individualising the drug treatment .

Proteomics investigation might represent a powerful holistic scientific approach in order to possibly characterised the molecular hallmarks of Neuroblastoma chemoresistance. Combining high-resolution protein separations with mass spectrometry protein identification, proteomics allows to explore the molecular mechanisms of cancer chemoresistance in a data driven experimental design, therefore enabling the construction of novel hypothesis not necessarily linked to a define researcher theory.

In the following the authors review the current state of the art in the proteomics investigations devoted to the characterisation of Neuroblastoma drug resistance.

Chapter III - Strikingly, Down syndrome (DS) or trisomy 21, protects against neuroblastoma. The authors aimed at understanding the mechanisms involved in this unique constitutional resistance to neural tumors. Indeed, an international epidemiological study conducted in 11 European countries did not find any case of neuroblastoma in children with DS among 6724 young children while more than five were expected [Satgé et al Cancer Research 1998;58:448-52]. Furthermore, only five cases of neuroblastic tumors have been reported so far in children with DS. The protective effect seems specific to peripheral neural tumors and also to central nervous system neural tumors such as medulloblastoma since, conversely, other cancers such as leukaemia, lymphoma, and germ cell tumors are more frequent in children with DS than in the general population. DS phenotype results from the genetic imbalance of the nearly 300 genes mapping to the supernumerary chromosome 21, theoretically up-regulated at a 150% rate through a gene dosage effect. As a matter of fact, adrenal medulla is frequently hypoplastic in children with DS. Several genes located on chromosome 21, expressed in neural and glial tissue may be involved in the reduced incidence of neuroblastoma. They play a role in various functions : apoptosis (ETS2, SOD1, APP), cellular adhesion via direct or indirect effect (DSCAM, CAR, APP), cellular proliferation (ANA, S100B, IFNGR2), anti-angiogenic activity (COL18A1, DSCR1, IFNAR1, IFNAR2, IFNGR2), cellular signalling (ETS2), neural cell maturation and differentiation (S100beta, TIAM1, APP).

We checked three different and complementary cellular approaches. First, *in vitro* growth of neuroblastoma cell lines IGR-N-91, SK-N-SH and SK-N-BE were inhibited by addition of S100B protein in the culture medium, and neuroblasts showed differentiation. Furthermore, the intratumoral injection of S100B in nude mice xenografted with the cell line IGR-N-91 resulted in a 5-10 fold tumor volume reduction compared to control mice. Second, differentiation of the SH-SY-5Y cell line with retinoic acid induced a PCP4 gene expression. Also, in the same cell line, only one additional copy of the PCP4 gene induced a more important and earlier differentiation of these tumoral neuroblasts. Third, the growth of SK-N-AS and SH-SY-5Y cell lines on an extra-cellular matrix (ECM) produced by trisomic 21 fibroblasts was reduced compared to euploid fibroblasts ECM.

These preliminary experiences provide tracks for understanding the striking constitutional resistance to NB in DS and highlight i) an over-maturation state of neural cells and/or ii), the role of extra-cellular molecules produced by Schwann cells and fibroblasts.

Chapter IV - In human neuroblastoma (NB), the wild-type (wt) p53 protein is retained in the cytoplasm of malignant neuroblasts, where it is unable to operate as a tumor suppressor in the nucleus. p73, the first homologue of the p53 gene, encodes a myriad of isoforms and variants due to alternative splicing at the NH2-

or COOH-terminal regions and alternative promoter usage. Two promoters have been described so far: P1, which encodes full-length TAp73α, and the cryptic promoter P2, which is located in intron 3 and produces ΔNp73α, an N-truncated variant lacking the transactivation domain. It has been shown that TAp73α can induce tumor suppressor properties such as cell-cycle arrest and apoptosis while ΔNp73α antagonizes the pro-apoptotic p53 in sympathetic neurons upon NGF withdrawal, thus acting as a dominant negative isoform. Data from previous studies of ours indicates that overexpressed TAp73 cooperates with wtp53 to induce apoptosis with high efficiency in wtp53 NB cells but not in mutated-p53 NB cells. This prompted us to postulate that TAp73 might be a candidate for neuronal differentiation, a biological process which hallmarks NB cells and is associated with specific protein expression. To explore this possibility, the authors infected two human NB cell lines, SH-SY5Y and IGR-N-91, with wtp53 and mutated p53, respectively, with TAp73alpha and ΔNp73α recombinant adenoviruses. cDNA macroarray analysis with the Atlas Human Cancer 1.2 Array (Clontech) showed that: i) TAp73α transactivated the expression of a number of genes associated with development and neuronal function, including Notch1, MIC-1/GDF-15, Jagged2, p75^{NTR} (NGFR), and chromogranin B in both cell lines; ii) ΔNp73α inhibited these developmental genes and repressed the S100 calcium-binding protein, known to be implicated in neuronal differentiation; iii) Wnt8A, known to be involved in development and neuronal differentiation, was only activated by TA-or ΔNp73 in SH-SY5Y cells, suggesting that transactivation in this case is not dependent on the NH2-terminal transactivation domain.

Chapter V - Neuroblastoma (NB), one of the common malignant childhood tumors, arises from neuroblast cells derived from the neural crest and destined for the adrenal medulla and the sympathetic nervous system and affects approximately 1 in 100,000 individuals. NB represents 7% to 10% of all malignancies diagnosed in pediatric patients younger than 15 years of age and is responsible for approximately 15% of all pediatric cancer deaths. However, NB is a heterogeneous disease; tumors can spontaneously regress or mature, or display a very aggressive, malignant phenotype. Because of these unique characteristics, NB has been of great interest to both clinicians and basic scientists. Progress in molecular and cellular biology and immunology in the past 10 years has contributed greatly to a better understanding of this disease; however, this progress has not significantly altered the clinical outcome for patients with NB. Cell apoptotic has been characterized by a progressive series of morphological and biochemical changes, it is a mechanism that organisms utilize to eliminate no need cells. Research shows the programmed cell death or apoptosis and its controlling gene abnormality is one of the main causes of tumor mechanism. Caspases protease families are Cysteinyl Aspartate Specific Protease (Caspase) plays a very important role in cancer apoptosis.

Chapter VI - Pediatric neuro-ectodermal tumors range from undifferentiated, truly malignant neuroblastomas, via ganglioneuroblastomas to well-differentiated, mostly benign ganglioneuromas. Within the group of malignant neuroblastomas, different risk categories can be identified: patients with high, intermediate or low risk tumors. High-risk tumors include disseminated disease or bulky tumors with gross genetic alterations, such as the amplification of the oncogene MYCN (INSS stages 3 and 4).

In: Neuroblastoma Research Trends
Editors: L. H. Andre and N. E. Roux
ISBN: 978-1-60456-790-8

Chapter I

Cancer Stem Cell in Neuroblastoma: Diagnostic and Therapeutic Implications

Hiroaki Komuro*
Department of Pediatric Surgery, Graduate School of Comprehensive Human Sciences, University of Tsukuba, Japan

Abstract

Neuroblastoma (NB) is a common pediatric solid tumor. Macroscopically as well as microscopically, NB shows a heterogeneous appearance. One important question is what the basis of this heterogeneity is. Another question is how this heterogeneity influences the biological characteristics and/or treatment strategy for NB. Recently, the first question has been well answered by the cancer stem cell theory. That is to say that cancer originates from a stem cell with the ability of self-renewal as well as multipotency. The cancer comprises a hierarchical organization with only a small number of cancer stem cells (CSCs) and a large number of their descendants. Only the CSCs are responsible for tumorigenicity, progression and metastasis in the cancer, while their descendants are not. Their descendants will differentiate, resulting in the heterogeneity of the cancer.

* Hiroaki Komuro, MD, PhD, 1-1-1 Tennodai, Tsukuba, Ibaraki 305-8575, Japan, TEL : +81-29-853-3094, FAX : +81-29-853-3149, E-mail : hiro-kom@md.tsukuba.ac.jp.

Recently, CSCs have been isolated from some cancers. The real target determining the biological characteristics and the treatment strategy should be the CSCs themselves instead of the rest (and the majority) of the constituent cancer cells. Normal stem cells and CSCs show similar resistance to current therapies, because they both stay in a quiescent state and have a common drug efflux capacity. This means that a small fraction of cancer stem cells can survive aggressive therapies, even though the remaining majority of the cancer cells are responsive to them. This eventually leads to relapse of the cancer. If this is the case with NB, isolation of the CSCs in NB is the first step for understanding their characteristics and for developing treatment strategies for them. Side population (SP) cells characterized by the efficient efflux of Hoechst 33342 dye are thought to be enriched for stem cells in many normal tissues. Recently, SP cells that showed stem cell characteristics were isolated from primary NB tumors as well as NB cell lines. We have also investigated SP cells in NB cell lines and found that NB cell lines contained a small fraction of SP cells. Furthermore, normal stem cells as well as CSCs are believed to be maintained by the microenvironment surrounding them (called the "niche"). It will be now important to focus on not only the small fraction of CSCs but also their niche in NB in order to characterize their biological behavior and to developing strategies to eradicate the tumor. A new era in neuroblastoma research has begun with the establishment of the cancer stem cell theory. The diagnostic and therapeutic implications of CSCs in NB are herein reviewed and discussed.

Introduction

Neuroblastoma (NB) is a common pediatric solid tumor which is derived from the neural crest. NB can be clinically divided into three risk groups [1]. One group of NB is a low-risk subset, and it sometimes regresses spontaneously, or differentiates to ganglioneuroblastoma or ganglioneuroma with age, presenting a good prognosis. In contrast, another is a high-risk subset and it is highly malignant and refractory to most treatments, presenting a poor prognosis. The remaining group constitutes an intermediate-risk subset. Patient age, tumor stage, pathologic findings, and some molecular markers have been considered to be associated with the biological behavior of NB [2-22]. The high-risk group of NB remains one of the most difficult childhood tumors to treat in spite of recent advances in multimodality therapies. At present, high-risk NB still poses a major challenge to clinical oncologists. It is clear that no conventional treatment strategy can eradicate high-risk NB. We have often experienced that although some NBs appeared to respond initially to aggressive treatments and became reduced in size, they restarted to progress later and finally relapsed. Some patients with apparently low-risk NB at diagnosis unexpectedly relapse and require more aggressive treatments. This suggests the possibility that some special fraction of cells in a given NB tissue will be refractory to treatments, whereas others will respond well to them. Actually the specimen of a NB tumor shows a heterogeneous appearance macroscopically as well as microscopically. Not all tumor cells in NB are likely to respond equally to a given treatment. Until now, however, researchers as well as clinicians have evaluated the biology of NB, while considering it to be relatively homogeneous, which is an assumption that can be justified when examining the bulk of a tumor. Recently overwhelming evidence supporting the cancer stem cell theory has been obtained for some cancers, including leukemia, brain tumors and breast cancers. If this theory could be applied to NB, not only the heterogeneity of NB but also its mechanism of relapse could be well explained.

Heterogeneity in Neuroblastoma

Recent studies have shown that carcinogenesis, in which a single normal cell is converted to a cancer cell, is a multistep process involving accumulated genetic as well as epigenetic alterations in key regulatory genes [23-24]. Cancer is believed to be a monoclonal population of cells arising from a single cell. If this were strictly the case, each cancer would consist of cells with a single phenotype, showing a rather homogeneous appearance (Figure 1). However, an actual cancer contains a variety of cells with different phenotypes. The heterogeneity (multiple phenotypes) observed in cancer is suggestive of an origin from a cell with multi-lineage potential. In solid tumors, irregularity of the shape and surface of tumors is highly suspicious of malignancy. The heterogeneity of the tumor is a rather good reflection of the malignancy. This is the case with NB. Malignant NB shows a heterogeneous appearance, whereas well-differentiated ganglioneuroma looks relatively homogeneous. When a NB tumor is removed at surgery, we are often at a loss to decide which part of the heterogeneous tumor should be submitted for pathological and biological examinations in order to make a correct diagnosis. Furthermore, when the tumor is removed after aggressive chemotherapies and/or radiotherapies, it contains a heterogeneous mixture of tissues, showing not only some viable portions but also other non-viable portions in the same tumor.

Certainly, not every cell in a NB tumor behaves in the same manner. NBs are thought to be derived from neural crest stem cells that are capable of multilineage differentiation. Microscopically, the NB tumor contains various kinds of neural crest-derived cells, including neuron-like cells, ganglion-like cells, Schwannian stromal cells and rare chromaffin cells. It also contains differentiated as well as undifferentiated cells. This heterogeneity characteristic of NB cannot be explained only by the multistep carcinogenesis theory (Figure 1).

Cancer Stem Cell Theory

Two general models of heterogeneity in solid tumor cells have been postulated [26]. In one, individual tumor cells of many different phenotypes each have the potential to proliferate and give rise to another tumor. In the other model, most tumor cells have only limited proliferative potential, while a subset of tumor cells can proliferate extensively and can form new tumors.

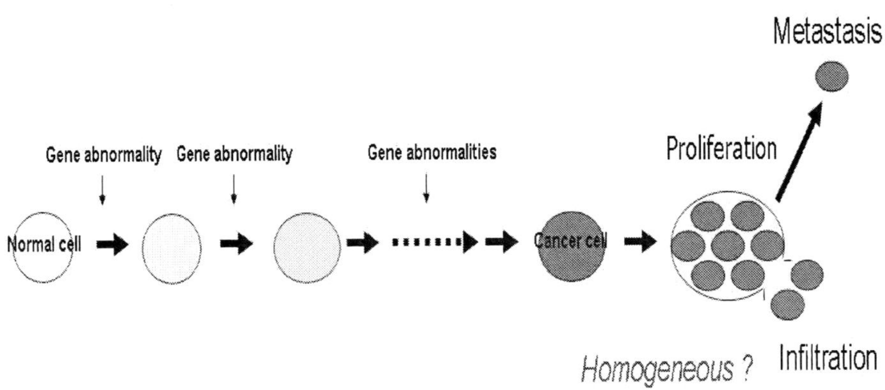

Figure 1. Multistep carcinogenesis model generally accepted for the development of cancer. Accumulation of multiple genetic abnormalities such as mutations and epigenetic changes drives a single cell to a cancer phenotype. In this model it is assumed that the resulting cancer is homogeneous. The heterogeneity of cancer cells cannot be explained only by this model.

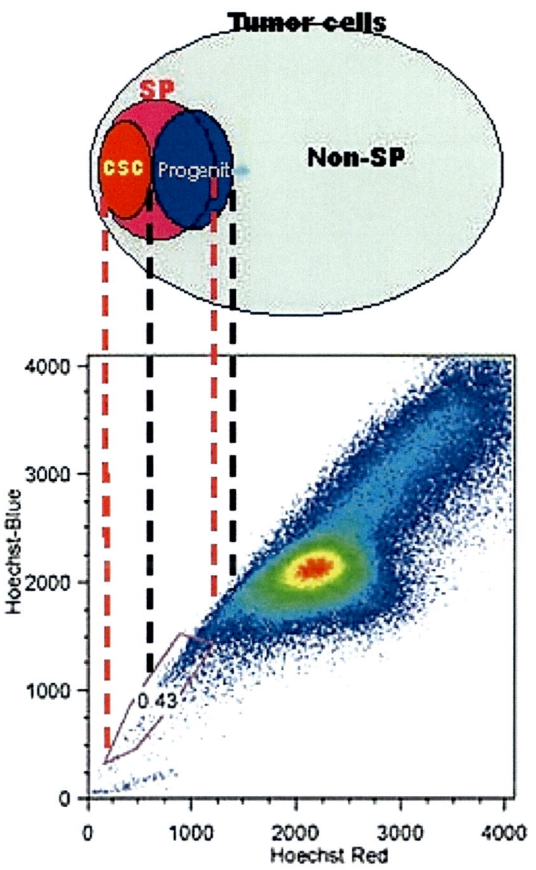

Figure 2. Side population (SP) cells were identified in a NB cell line. SP cells may be enriched in the cancer stem cells, but may contain stem-like cancer cells with different phenotypes, including a population of progenitor cells. CSC, cancer stem cell; SP, side population.

On the other hand, many previous studies have shown that, in a variety of hematological and solid tumors, more than 10^2-10^6 murine and human tumor cells are required to reproduce a new tumor and that only a few cells (less than 1-4%) within a tumor can form new tumors [27-34]. This subset of tumor cells have been called tumor-initiating cells (TICs). Considering these results, the latter model is rather more reasonable. If this is true, this subset would have not only the potential to form new tumors (tumorigenicity), but also the potential to produce the heterogeneity. Results supporting this model were first reported in acute myeloid leukemia (AML). Lapidot et al. demonstrated that only a small subset of human AML cells that were phenotypically similar to normal hematopoietic stem cells could produce AML when transplanted into immunodeficient mice. Other AML cells were unable to induce leukemia [35]. This indicates that AML cells are intrinsically heterogeneous in their proliferative potential, and that a small subset of AML stem cells gives rise to a much larger population of leukemia cells that lack the ability to proliferate extensively. This strongly supported the cancer stem cell theory, i.e., the idea that cancer develops from tissue stem cells (Figure 3). A stem cell is a cell that has the potential of self-renewal and multipotency. A stem cell is quiescent most of the time, and it occasionally divides asymmetrically, producing itself that retains its stem cell properties and a daughter cell that differentiates into a particular phenotype. A constant overall number of stem cells is maintained by strict regulation. Stem cells have a long life span and are self-renewing (undergoing repeated DNA synthesis), while progenitor or mature cells have a limited life span. This implies that multiple gene abnormalities, including mutations and epigenetic changes, are more likely to accumulate in stem cells than in progenitors and mature cells. Accordingly, cancer can be generated by the CSCs as a result of the deregulation of self-renewal in stem cells (Figure 3). In addition to reproducing themselves, the CSCs can also generate their descendants, including rapidly growing progenitor cells and relatively differentiated cancer cells, and thereby generate heterogeneity of the cancer (Figure 3). The CSCs are expected to retain the properties common to normal stem cells.

Special properties, including self-renewal, multipotency and asymmetrical division, that normal stem cells have are called “stemness”. Interestingly, some genes maintaining “stemness” have been shown to be the same as the genes involved in carcinogenesis [36-42]. The oncogenic pathway is closely related to the pathways maintaining self-renewal and differentiation in stem cells. A cancer cell is more likely to originate from a stem cell with deregulated self-renewal. The common signaling pathways in carcinogenesis and stemness include Bmi1, Wnt, Hedgehog, and Notch signaling pathways. These signaling pathways are well known to be deregulated in a variety of cancers. Polycomb transcription repressor Bmi1 plays an important role in embryogenesis as well as in the prevention of senescence, apoptosis and possibly differentiation in stem cells [42]. It acts on cell cycle progression through p16 inhibition and represses apoptosis through p19^{arf}/p53. Overexpression of Bmi1 leads to the development of cancers including leukemia, medulloblastoma, and breast cancer [37, 43-45]. Deregulation of Bmi1 signaling pathways associated with stemness appears to contribute to the development of a variety of cancers [37-38,43-46]. Wnt signaling through β-catenin influences the proliferation and renewal of stem cells or progenitor cells during the development of tissues. Deregulated activation of Wnt/β-catenin signaling is associated with the formation of a variety of cancers through the activation of gene transcription by β-catenin [39-40,47-49]. This pathway also plays an important role in both neural proliferation and neuronal differentiation as well as in neural crest stem cell maintenance [50-53]. Hedgehog (HH), which plays an important role in embryonic development, has been also shown to also be a stem cell regulator that promotes the differentiation of both embryonal and adult stem cells [39-42, 54-55]. HH signaling is mediated by Smoothened/Patched receptor complex. Activating mutations in Smoothened or inactivation of Patched have been shown to be responsible for some cancers such as basal cell carcinoma, brain tumors, prostate cancers and gastrointestinal tumors, as well as some birth defects [55-59]. Aberrant activation of HH signaling downstream elements such as Gli has also been shown to be associated with the development of various cancers [55, 58, 60]. Notch is crucial for the maintenance and differentiation (change of structure and function) of stem cells during fetal and postnatal development. The Notch family of receptors has been implicated in the self-renewal of tissues in organs such as the skin, the gut and the hematopoietic system. Stem cell maintenance, cell fate decisions and the initiation of cell differentiation are controlled by Notch signaling. Deregulation of these functions leads to tumorigenesis [61-68]. Thus, "stemness" genes have been shown to be strongly associated with cancer development. This strongly supports the cancer stem cell theory.

The CSCs resemble normal stem cells morphologically as well as immunohistochemi-cally in AML, in which CSCs were first identified [35]. The CSCs are believed to retain the properties similar to those of normal stem cells. As normal tissues are maintained by a small fraction of stem cells which can produce themselves as well as tissue constituent cells simultaneously, cancer is also maintained by a hierarchical organization composed of a small fraction of CSCs responsible for tumorigenesis and a majority of their descendants. There is accumulating evidence that cancer contains a minor fraction of CSCs in addition to the major fraction consisting of their descendants, including rapidly proliferating and differentiating progenitor cells and relatively differentiated cancer cells. Cancer also contains cells derived from other tissues, such as bone marrow-derived stem cells which contribute to angiogenesis. Both endogenous and exogenous stem cells contribute to the development and maintenance of cancer. This hierarchical organization provides more complicated heterogeneity of the cancer, although the heterogeneity seems to be mostly due to the multipotency of the CSCs themselves. Although it is difficult to determine

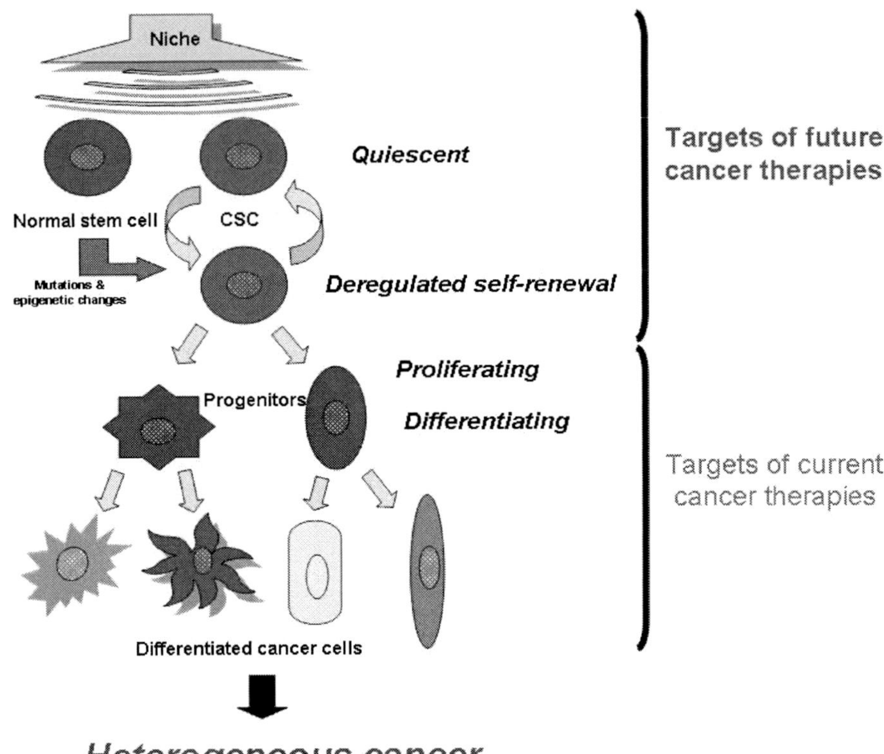

Figure 3. Schema showing cancer stem cell theory and new therapeutic strategies based on it. CSC, cancer stem cell.

whether the unlimited proliferation of cancer is due to deregulation of self-renewal in stem cells, or whether it is due to the acquisition of stemness properties by mature cells, increasing evidence has supported the former. Only a small fraction of CSCs have the potential for tumorigenicity, progression andmetastasis like TICs, whereas the large majority of cancer constituent cells do not. Furthermore, CSCs and normal stem cells are considered to show similar drug resistance. The CSCs appear to be resistant to conventional therapies in the same way as normal stem cells, and they can survive aggressive therapies that can eliminate the rest of the cancer cells. Finally, this is followed by relapse of the cancer after a temporary remission. The real target for eradicating cancer should be therefore the CSCs themselves. Accordingly, it is now time to change our way of thinking about cancer and to design new therapeutic strategies on the basis of the cancer stem cell theory.

Tumorigenesis of NB and Cancer Stem Cells

NB derives from neural crest stem cells during embryogenesis. The neural crest is a transient, highly migratory population of multipotent cells that give rise to the neurons and glia of the sympathetic nervous system and other diverse cell types such as melanocytes, enteric neurons, sensory neurons and cranial cartilage. NBs are thought to be derived from the neural crest cells with sympathetic nervous system differentiation fate. The neural crest represents one of the most dramatic examples of stem or progenitor cell heterogeneity [69]. It is not surprising that the tumors arising from a stem cell population that is highly migratory and simultaneously proliferating give rise to the most aggressive form of NB. However, in contrast, a subset of NBs show favorable prognosis with a tendency to differentiation or regression. Accordingly, Nakagawara postulated that there are two different types of NB stem cells [70]. One type of NBs derived from cancer stem cells of type A have a favorable prognosis and are characterized by high expression of TrkA and p75NTR and dependence on NGF. They occur in both sympathetic ganglia and adrenal medulla and have mitotic dysfunction, showing hyperdiploidy. The other type of NBs are derived from cancer stem cells of type B and are localized in the adrenal medulla. They have an unfavorable prognosis and are prone to have genetic instability that causes *MYCN* amplification and allelic loss of chromosome 1p36. They may retain rather immature phenotypes with diploid karyotype, expressing not TrkA but TrkB [70]. Probably CSCs generated from specific stem cells at various stages during the development of the sympathetic nervous system may be responsible for the tumorigenesis of NB.

Exposure to environmental toxins is probably not a major cause of NB or of some other pediatric tumors. Genes that are often mutated in adult tumors, such as p53, p16, p19, p27, and NF1, are rarely disrupted in NB [71-72]. Childhood tumors are fundamentally different from adult cancers, both in their cells of origin and possibly in the genetic lesions that lead to malignancy. The development of NB is strongly related to embryogenesis. Recent studies have shown that the abnormalities in some "stemness" genes which also contribute to embryogenesis are associated with the tumorigenesis of NB. Bmi1 is strongly expressed in NB and is associated with tumorigenesis as a target of E2F-1 proteins, which also regulate *MYCN* gene expression [73]. Recently, attention has been paid to the involvement of Wnt-5a through Wnt/β-calcium signaling in the pathogenesis of NB [74-75]. The Notch pathway may also be involved in the tumorigenesis of NB and play a role in promoting the development of dedifferentiated phenotypes. Under hypoxic conditions, the Notch cascade is activated, and might promote the development of the dedifferentiated (more malignant) phenotype of NB [76-77]. Further studies may clarify the roles of the "stemness" genes in the CSCs of NB.

Attempts to Isolate Cancer Stem Cells from NB

The next important step in understanding the fundamental biology of a cancer and furthermore in eliminating it is to identify the CSCs. The CSCs derived from deregulated tissue stem cells are expected to share the similar properties with normal stem cells. That means that CSCs may be isolated by the same procedures as those used to isolate tissue stem cells. Recent studies have shown that only a small subset of tumor cells in an existing tumor have tumor-initiating potential, and that this subset of cells also have the functional properties (self-renewal and differentiation potential) that normal stem cells share. These stem-like cancer cells are considered to be the CSCs. The big problems in isolating normal stem cells as well as CSCs are their rarity and the absence of specific markers for purifying them. Several efforts have been made to isolate CSCs from various cancers. The CSCs were first identified in AML as TICs that could reproduce the original cancer with heterogeneous phenotypes and expressed the stem cell surface markers CD34+,CD38- [35]. To date, the CSCs or stem-like cancer cells have been isolated mainly as side population (SP) cells that export Hoechst 33342 dye, a fraction of cancer cells expressing specific cell surface markers, and cancer cells that form spheres.

1. Identification of Side Population (SP) Cells in NB

Recently a low-abundance fraction of side population (SP) cells has been focused on as a fraction which contains stem cells. SP cells are characterized by rapid efflux of Hoechst 33342 dye via the ATP binding cassette (ABC) transporter, as shown by fluorescence-activated cell sorter (FACS) analysis. It has been shown that stem cells are enriched in SP cells in various normal tissues, including bone marrow, skeletal muscle, mammary gland, skin, lung, testis, brain, liver, and kidney [78-86]. Transcriptional profiling studies of SP and non-SP cells in several tissues showed that the genes upregulated in SP cells are implicated in the quiescent status, the maintenance of pluripotency and the capacity to undergo asymmetric division [87]. SP cells have also been identified in several tumor cell lines as well as fresh tumor samples, including NB [88-92]. Hirschmann-Jax et al. demonstrated that SP cells were found to constitute 0.8-51% of the cells in 15 of 23 NB tumor samples as well as 4-37% of the cells in five NB cell lines. SP cells in NB were Gd2+, c-kit+, CD133-, CD71-, CD56± and expressed ABC transporter proteins ABCG2 and ABCA3 at high levels, supporting the possibility that they were CSCs [88]. We have also examined the SP fraction in several NB cell lines using FACS analysis and identified SP cells in all NB cell lines examined (Figure 2). Unlike fresh tumor samples, cell lines do not contain any contaminating non-cancer stem cells such as bone marrow-derived stem cells. Accordingly, the SP cells identified in cell lines are definitely derived from cancer cells. It was expected that NB stem cells might be enriched in the SP fraction. The SP cells in NB may be considered a stem-like population, but may not always be pure stem cell themselves. ABC transporter proteins, whose expression is characteristic of SP cells, may be intimately involved not only in the biology of stem cells but also in that of progenitor cells. Thus, SP cells may contain progenitor cells as well as stem cells. Since the gate used for the SP fraction in the dual wavelength analysis shows a wide range of area, some SP cells are located very close to and others are far from non-SP cells. This may imply that the SP cells may be composed of a rather heterogeneous population. It is reasonable that the SP cells in NB may include not only stem cells but also some progenitor cells (Figure 2). There is a possibility that the SP fraction might contain quiescent stem cells as well as rapidly growing precursor cells. Further analysis may be required to examine this possibility.

2. Identification of Cancer Stem Cells Using Specific Cell Surface Markers

In some cancers, organ-specific stem cell surface markers have also been identified and used to purify CSCs. CSCs were first identified in AML. Only a small fraction of CD34+, CD38- cells possess leukemia initiating capacity, while the large majority of CD34+, CD38+ and CD34- cells in the cancer do not [35]. Brain cancer stem cells were isolated by FACS using neural stem cell surface marker CD133. These CD133+ cells self-renewed and differentiated into tumor cells similarly to the original tumor [93]. Breast cancer stem cells were isolated using CD44+, CD24-, Lineage- cells [94], which were associated with normal ductal stem cells. A small number of these sorted cells could not only cause tumorigenesis, but could also self-renew and generate non-tumorigenic cancer cells. Although cell surface markers expressed in neural crest stem cells may be useful for isolating NB stem cells, no specific markers for NB stem cells have been identified yet. Neural crest stem cells can produce cells with a variety of phenotypes, including melanocytes, sensory neurons, enteric neurons and sympathetic ganglion cells. The fact that NB never occurs in tissues other than sympathetic ganglion and adrenal medulla suggests that the genetic events that cause NB occur after the cell fate determination directing cells toward sympathetic nervous system differentiation. Many important genes regulating normal differentiation of the sympathetic nervous system have been targeted in an attempt to cause NB. Further studies will be required to identify the key regulatory markers in NB stem cells.

3. Morphological Identification of Cancer Stem Cells

Morphological characterization can be used to isolate the CSCs. Sphere formation was used for isolating CSCs in some cancers. The formation of neurospheres and mammospheres are characteristic of neural and mammary stem cells [95-96]. Such sphere formation was also observed in brain tumor and breast cancer cells, respectively. Tumor-derived neurospheres found in pediatric brain tumors showed characteristics similar to neural stem cells as well as tumorigenic potential [97]. Nonadherent mammospheres have been shown to be enriched in early progenitor/stem cells. Using this technique of mammosphere formation, the CSCs in breast cancers were isolated [98]. It has been suggested that cells with the morphological characteristics of the CSCs are present in NB [99-101]. There are three types of NB phenotypes among the cells found in human NB cell lines. N-type cells are the most common sympathoadrenal neuroblasts, which grow as poorly attached aggregates of small rounded cells with short neuritic processes. A second type of cells, S-type cells, resemble non-neuronal precursor cells, and attach strongly to the substrate as large flattened cells, showing contact inhibition of cell growth. A third type, I-type cells, show the morphological and growth characteristics intermediate between those of N and S types. I-type cells form aggregates in culture and are recognized as malignant NB stem cells based on their unique differentiation and malignant potentials [99-100]. Whereas N- and S-type cells appear to be progenitors committed to a specific differentiation, I-type cells are less differentiated and have greater phenotypic stability, are capable of bidirectional differentiation to N- and S-type cells in the presence of inducers and are strongly tumorigenic [101-102]. However, these three types of cells can not be clearly defined morphologically even if combined immunohistochemical examinations are applied. I-type cells express neural stem cell marker Nestin and stem cell marker proteins CD133 and c-kit [102]. On the other hand, SP cells from NB express c-kit but not CD133 [88]. Continued efforts to search for specific NB stem cell markers will be required.

Resistance of Cancer Stem Cells to Current Therapies

A subset of cancer cells in the tumor may be more resistant to therapy than the other cells. Conventional cancer therapies have been designed to kill rapidly dividing cells as a target. If the CSCs do originate from normal stem cells and have similarities of drug resistance, it is important to know the mechanism of drug resistance in normal stem cells. Two mechanisms are assumed to underlie the therapeutic resistance which CSCs and normal stem cells share.

1. Cancer Stem Cells may be Quiescent and Rarely Dividing

Normal stem cells may lie dormant in G0 of the cell cycle and divide relatively infrequently, staying in a quiescent state, whereas their descendants, including progenitors and more differentiated cells, divide rather rapidly to produce many progeny. Presumably, the CSCs may also stay quiescent in the same way as normal stem cells, whereas the remaining descendant cells show progressive expansion and differentiate during progression through the cell cycle. As a result, the tumor contains a heterogeneous collection of cells consisting of a minor fraction of quiescent CSCs and a majority of cancer constituent cells (proliferating progenitor cells and partially differentiated cancer cells). Although the majority of cancer constituent cells are responsive to current therapies which target rapidly dividing cells, the minor fraction of CSCs can survive in a quiescent state for many years after remission. They can then re-proliferate and cause relapse or metastasis later. Conventional treatments will be ineffective for the CSCs in a quiescent state.

2. Cancer Stem Cells Express ABC Transporters

It is well known that some cancer cells can survive anti-cancer drugs due to their resistance to these drugs. A variety of ATP binding cassette (ABC) transporters, including multiple drug resistance protein (MDR1, ABCB1), MDR related protein (MRP1, ABCC1), and breast cancer resistant protein (BRCP1, ABCG2), have been shown to contribute to the drug resistance in cancers [103-107]. Interestingly, some of these ABC transporters are also expressed in various kinds of normal stem cells [108-109]. This suggests that the CSCs have drug resistance due to expression of the same transporters. BRCP1 (ABCG2) is known to contribute to the exclusion of Hoechst 33342 dye in SP cells which are enriched in stem cells [109]. In other words, SP cells are partially characterized by BRCP expression. ABCG2 expressed in normal stem cells and CSCs is believed to play a physiological role in the protection of stem cells. In NB, the SP cells showed high expression of ABCG2 and ABCA3 [88]. Although some ABC transporters, including ABCB1 and ABCC1, are known to be related to drug resistance in NB [110-113], the roles of ABCG2 and ABCA3 in the drug resistance of NB have yet to be examined.

Therapeutic Implications of Cancer Stem Cells: New Strategies for Eradicating Cancer Stem Cells (Figure 3)

Conventional treatments have targeted the rapidly growing cancer cells, which are synthesizing DNA. In other words, the target of these treatments is not the CSC but the rest of the cancer-constituent cells. New treatment strategies for targeting the CSCs will be required to eradicate the cancer completely (Figure 3). To accomplish this, it is important to understand the mechanism of self-renewal in normal stem cells and its deregulation in CSCs. Possibly, how to attack only the CSCs selectively without any influence on the normal tissue stem cells will be a difficult problem.

1. Inhibitors of Signaling Pathways Deregulated in Cancer Stem Cells

The uncontrplled self-renewal of the CSCs may be maintained by deregulation of specific signaling pathways associated with stemness in normal stem cells. Inhibition of these deregulated pathways will be an effective treatment strategy, although it may be difficult to attack only CSCs without interfering with normal stem cells. There have been several reports on the application of specific inhibitors of these pathways to cancer therapies. Selective anti-Wnt antibodies, Wnt protein inhibitors such as WIF-1 or repressors disrupting nuclear LEF/TCF/b-catenin complexes may be effective for tumor growth inhibition [114-117]. Inhibitors of hedgehog signaling pathways have also been developed and applied to some cancers such as medulloblastoma [117-121]. Notch signaling inhibitors may be promising for the control of some cancers [122-123]. In the future it will be necessary to evaluate the effects of these signaling pathway inhibitors on the CSCs in order to eradicate the cancers.

2. Inhibitors of ABC Transporters

Normal stem cells as well as CSCs show similar drug resistance that is dependent on ABC transporter proteins that actively export anti-cancer drugs. This has led to the idea that ABC transporter inhibitors may be effective for eradicating the CSCs. Many drugs such as the calcium channel blocker verapamil and the immunosuppressant cyclosporin A have been shown to inhibit anti-cancer drug resistance by functioning as competitive substrates of MDR. Several efforts toward clinical application of these inhibitors have been made, but unfortunately they failed to obtain promising results [124-125]. The main problem related to these first-generation inhibitors was that they generally showed weak effects and strong toxicity at resistance-inhibiting doses. The second-generation inhibitors, which include PSC-833, VX-710, LY335979, XR9051 and XR9576, are in the process of being tested clinically [126-130]. The development of inhibitors of ABCG2, which is expressed in normal stem cells as well as SP cells enriched in CSCs, has been strongly anticipated [108-109]. These include GF120918 [131], XR9576 [132] and tRA98006 [133]. The development of novel inhibitors of ABC transporters which CSCs use may be an important step toward eradicating the CSCs. However, Patrawala et al. recently demonstrated that ABCG2+ and ABCG2- cells in several cancers showed a similar tumorigenic potential, although

SP cells are enriched in tumorigenic, stem-like cancer cells [134]. Further studies may be required to clarify the relationship between SP cells and their expression of ABC transporters other than ABCG2 and the relationship between SP cells and tumorigenic CSCs.

3. Monoclonal Antibodies to Cell Surface Markers on Cancer Stem Cells

Monoclonal antibody to CD33 on the surface of AML blasts has been applied to patients with relapsed CD33-positive AML [135]. If the CSCs show specific cell surface markers, developing monoclonal antibodies that recognize them may be one of the treatment choices.

4. Differentiation Therapies

Since CSCs are considered to retain the potential for multi-lineage differentiation, differentiation therapy will be a promising strategy for the management of CSCs. In NB, a subset with favorable prognosis is known to regress or differentiate spontaneously. To date, it has been demonstrated that some differentiation inducers, such as retinoic acid, phorbolester and NGF, can promote the differentiation or apoptosis of some NB cells [136-141]. Ross et al. demonstrated that I-type cells, which were thought to be a candidate of NB stem cells showed a capacity for differentiation into other types of cells [99,102]. These findings may suggest that differentiation therapy may provide better results for the management of the CSCs in NB. Another factor influencing the differentiation of NB is hypoxia. Hypoxic conditions may shift NB cells toward an immature stem-like phenotype through dedifferentiation [142-145]. As the CSCs are considered to be resistant to hypoxia like normal stem cells, hypoxia may contribute to the survival of the CSCs in NB. Further studies on the effects of hypoxia on CSCs will provide another differentiation treatment strategy for NB. If the CSCs in NB responsible for tumorigenesis, progression and metastasis are identified, induction of their differentiation could be one of the most effective treatments. To accomplish this, it will be required that the newly developed drugs not only force the CSCs to differentiate but also block their capacity of self-renewal. This will result in complete removal of the CSC pool as a reservoir of cancer cells.

Diagnostic Implications of CSCs in NB

Tumor samples contain a mixture of non-neoplastic and neoplastic cells, including immune cells, inflammatory cells, vascular endothelial cells, stromal cells, non-tumorigenic cancer cells, cancer progenitor cells and CSCs. For a correct diagnosis, the samples are subjected to pathological and biological examinations such as morphological, immunohisto-chemical, and molecular analyses. However, until now, they have been evaluated mainly on the basis of the characteristics of the majority of the cancer constituent cells. This is especially the case with biological examinations, because the samples are processed using the bulk of the tumor. Here, we should note that the most important sample for diagnostic and prognostic evaluations is the rare fraction of CSCs, not the main population of heterogeneous cancer constituent cells. The cancer stem cell theory has opened a new era in cancer research. The identification, isolation and characterization of CSCs will lead to correct diagnoses as well as correct assessments of prognosis. Evaluation of expression profiles and molecular signaling pathways in the CSCs will provide a new useful system for classification of cancers. In the near future, NB should be classified according to the characteristics of the CSCs.

Oncogenic Implications of CSCs in NB: Development and Cancer

The regulatory genes involved in embryonal development (e.g., Bmi1, Wnt/β-catenin, Notch, Hedgehog) play an important role in maintaining embryonic as well as adult stem cells. Deregulation of these genes leads to the development of cancer. Dean et al. called cancer a "developmental disorder", because it involves a disruption of normal development with respect to not only differentiation but also proliferation [146]. Many known oncogenes and tumor suppressor genes are involved in these embryonic regulatory gene pathways. NB is considered o be a tumor which arises during embryogenesis. Research on the molecular mechanism of the maintenance and differentiation of neural crest stem cells during embryogenesis and its deregulation (the CSCs in NB) is important not only for understanding sympathetic nervous system development, but also for understanding and treating NB.

To date, *MYCN* amplification is the strongest malignant marker in NB. Recent studies demonstrated that *MYCN* amplification does not appear to be associated with stem cell properties in NB, because it is not related to the SP subset in NB or to I-type cells [88,101]. The significance of *MYCN* amplification in the development of the CSCs in NB should be investigated in future studies.

Future Directions: Cancer Stem Cells and Stem Cell Niche

The microenvironment that stem cells reside in is called the "niche". The niche exerts important effects on cellular phenotypes as well as their maintenance in normal stem cells. The surrounding components, including stromal cells, extracellular matrix, and microvessels, are considered to constitute a stem cell niche. If CSCs are derived from tissue stem cells, the CSC niche may also play an important role in tumorigenesis, tumor progression and tumor maintenance. Stem cell behavior or fate is determined by the surrounding niche. Yamashita et al. demonstrated that interaction between stem cells and niche cells may be important in deciding that stem cells will create more copies of themselves after asymmetrical division. Otherwise, the other cells which are detached from niche cells differentiate into several phenotypes [147]. The special balanced interaction of stem cells and their surrounding niche may play an essential role in maintaining the homeostasis of stem cells. This balanced regulation of stem cells by the niche may strongly contribute to preventing tumorigenesis. If this is true, defects of the niche might be capable of giving rise to cancer. Tumorigenesis due to the development of the CSCs may involve the deregulation or alteration of their surrounding niche (Figure 3). Furthermore, interaction between the CSCs and their surrounding niche may play an important role in not only tumorigenesis but also tumor progression or differentiation fate. Recently it was reported that the onset of breast cancer may be caused by defects of somatic stem cell niches [148]. Myoepithelial cells comprising a niche have been shown to play a key role in breast cancer progression [149]. Previously, such stromal cells were ignored as a less-important factor in breast cancer. The stromal cells and extracellular matrices comprising the niche in a tumor have received little attention from many oncologists and pathologists. In NB, however, the direct correlation of abundant Schannian stroma with a favorable prognosis and with tumor maturation has been emphasized, suggesting the functional interaction between neuroblasts and the

Schwannian stroma [7-8]. Although Schwann cells do not belong to the neoplastic population, they are likely not only to be recruited from the surrounding tissue by neoplastic neuronal cells but also to be involved in the differentiation of NB cells in response to the expression of neurotrophic factors [150]. Recently, Liu et al. demonstrated that cross-talk between Schwann cells and neuroblasts could modify the biology of NB in a xenotransplant model [151]. In that study, infiltrating Schwann cells of mouse origin changed the biology of xenotransplanted human NB from an unfavorable to a favorable phenotype. Although the origin of Schwann cells remains controversial [150, 152-153], they are capable of influencing the phenotypes of NB and producing angiogenesis inhibitors or neurotrophic factors [153-157]. Another component of the niche is a specialized microvascular bed of endothelial cells derived from bone marrow-derived stem cells. This plays an important role in supplying some nutrients as well as oxygen to the stem cells. Hypoxia may influence the characteristics and proliferation of normal stem cells and CSCs, as they can thrive under hypoxia [142-145,158-160]. In the near future, investigation of the interaction between stem cells and their niche will lead to a better understanding of the mechanisms of the development, invasiveness, and metastasis of cancers, including NB. Furthermore, targeting not neoplastic cells but their surrounding niche will provide a new treatment strategy for NB (Figure 3). The status of the CSCs is maintained by the surrounding "niche". Although the origin of NB stem cells remains unknown so far, future studies to clarify the roles of the CSCs as well as the stem cell niche in NB development will be important. These efforts will enable us to understand the mechanism of the development of NB during embryogenesis as well as to develop novel treatment strategies to eradicate NB. These efforts may also answer the questions of why the biology of NB depends on age, or why some NBs behave aggressively despite current therapies, and others less aggressively.

In summary, as the cancer stem cell theory has opened the new windows in cancer research, it is time to change our way of thinking about cancer. More attention should be paid to two important components involved in cancer that are responsible for the development, progression and maintenance of cancer. One is a minor population of the CSCs which operates as a reservoir of cancer cells. The other is the surrounding niche, which maintains the CSCs. Targeting these two components will provide a new treatment strategy to eradicate cancers completely.

References

[1] Castleberry RP, Pritchard J, Ambros P, Berthold F, Brodeur GM, Castel V, Cohn SL, De Bernardi B, Dicks-Mireaux C, Frappaz D, Haase GM, Haber M, Jones DR, Joshi VV, Kaneko M, Kemshead JT, Kogner P, Lee RE, Matthay KK, Michon JM, Monclair R, Roald BR, Seeger RC, Shaw PJ, Shuster JJ (1997) The International Neuroblastoma Risk Groups (INRG): a preliminary report. *Eur. J. Cancer* 33:2113-2116.

[2] Breslow N, McCann B. (1971) Statistical estimation of prognosis for children with neuroblastoma. *Cancer Res.* 31:2098–2103.

[3] Brodeur GM, Azar C, Brother M, Hiemstra J, Kaufman B, Marshall H, Moley J, Nakagawara A, Saylors R, Scavarda N (1992) Neuroblastoma. Effect of genetic factors on prognosis and treatment. *Cancer* 70: 1685-1694.

[4] Evans AE, D'Angio GJ, Randolph J. (1971) A proposed staging for children with neuroblastoma. Children's Cancer Study Group A. *Cancer* 27:374–378.

[5] Evans AE, D'Angio GJ, Propert K, Anderson J, Hann HW.(1987) Prognostic factors in neuroblastoma. *Cancer* 59:1853–1859.

[6] Brodeur GM, Pritchard J, Berthold F, Carlsen NL, Castel V, Castelberry RP, De Bernardi B, Evans AE, Favrot M, Hedborg F (1993) Revisions of the international criteria for neuroblastoma diagnosis, staging, and response to treatment. *J. Clin. Oncol.* 11: 1466-1477.

[7] Shimada H, Ambros IM, Dehner LP, Hata J, Joshi VV, Roald B, Stram DO, Gerbing RB, Lukens JN, Matthay KK, Castleberry RP. (1999) The International Neuroblastoma Pathology Classification (the Shimada system). *Cancer* 86: 364-372.

[8] Shimada H, Umehara S, Monobe Y, Hachitanda Y, Nakagawa A, Goto S, Gerbing RB, Stram DO, Lukens JN, Matthay KK. (2001) International neuroblastoma pathology classification for prognostic evaluation of patients with peripheral neuroblastic tumors: a report from the Children's Cancer Group. *Cancer* 92: 2451-2461.

[9] Brodeur GM, Seeger RC, Schwab M, Varmus HE, Bishop JM. (1984) Amplification of N-*myc* in untreated human neuroblastomas correlates with advanced disease stage. *Science* 224:1121–1124.

[10] Seeger RC, Brodeur GM, Sather H, Dalton A, Siegel SE, Wong KY, Hammond D. (1985) Association of multiple copies of the N-*myc* oncogene with rapid progression of neuroblastomas. *N. Engl. J. Med.* 313:1111–1116.
[11] Look AT, Hayes FA, Nitschke R, McWilliams NB, Green AA. (1984) Cellular DNA content as a predictor of response to chemotherapy in infants with unresectable neuroblastoma. *N. Engl. J. Med.* 311:231–235.
[12] Look AT, Hayes FA, Shuster JJ, Douglass EC, Castleberry RP, Bowman LC, Smith EI, Brodeur GM. (1991) Clinical relevance of tumor cell ploidy and N-*myc* gene amplification in childhood neuroblastoma: a Pediatric Oncology Group study. *J. Clin. Oncol.* 9:581–591.
[13] Maris JM, Matthay KK. (1999) Molecular biology of neuroblastoma. *J. Clin. Oncol.* 17: 2264–2279.
[14] Guo C, White PS, Weiss MJ, Hogarty MD, Thompson PM, Stram DO, Gerbing R, Matthay KK, Seeger RC, Brodeur GM, Maris JM. (1999) Allelic deletion at 11q23 is common in *MYCN* single copy neuroblastomas. *Oncogene* 18:4948–4957.
[15] Thompson PM, Seifried BA, Kyemba SK, Jensen SJ, Guo C, Maris JM, Brodeur GM, Stram DO, Seeger RC, Gerbing R, Matthay KK, Matise TC, White PS. (2001) Loss of heterozygosity for chromosome 14q in neuroblastoma. *Med. Pediatr. Oncol.* 36:28–31.
[16] Caron H, van Sluis P, de Kraker J, Bokkerink J, Egeler M, Laureys G, Slater R, Westerveld A, Voute PA, Versteeg R. (1996) Allelic loss of chromosome 1p as a predictor of unfavorable outcome in patients with neuroblastoma. *N. Engl. J. Med.* 334: 225–230.
[17] Maris JM, White PS, Beltinger CP, Sulman EP, Castleberry RP, Shuster JJ, Look AT, Brodeur GM. (1995) Significance of chromosome 1p loss of heterozygosity in neuroblastoma. *Cancer Res.* 55:4664–4669.
[18] Nakagawara A, Arima M, Azar CG Scavarda NJ, Brodeur GM. (1992) Inverse relationship between *trk* expression and N-*myc* amplification in human neuroblastomas. *Cancer Res.* 52:1364–1368.
[19] Nakagawara A, Arima-Nakagawara M, Scavarda NJ, Azar CG, Cantor AB, Brodeur GM. (1993) Association between high levels of expression of the *TRK* gene and favorable outcome in human neuroblastoma. *N. Engl. J. Med.* 328:847–854.
[20] Ryden M, Sehgal R, Dominici C, Schilling FH, Ibanez CF, Kogner P. (1996) Expression of mRNA for the neurotrophin receptor trkC in neuroblastomas with favourable tumour stage and good prognosis. *Br. J. Cancer* 74:773–779.

[21] Yamashiro DJ, Nakagawara A, Ikegaki N, Liu XG, Brodeur GM. (1996) Expression of *TrkC* in favorable human neuroblastomas. *Oncogene* 12:37–41.

[22] Nakagawara A, Azar CG, Scavarda NJ, Brodeur GM. (1994) Expression and function of *TRK*-B and BDNF in human neuroblastomas. *Mol. Cell Biol.* 14:759–767.

[23] Robertson M (1983) Oncogenes and multistep carcinogenesis. *Br. Med. J.* (Clin Res Ed). 287:1084-1086.

[24] Land H, Parada LF, Weinberg RA (1993) Cellular oncogenes and multistep carcinogenesis. *Science* 222:771-778.

[25] Vogelstein, B. and K. W. Kinsler. (1993) The multistep nature of cancer. *Trends in Genetics* 9:138-141.

[26] Reya T, Morrison SJ, Clarke MF, Weissman IL. (2001) Stem cells, cancer, and cancer stem cells. *Nature* 414:105-111.

[27] Park CH, Bergsagel DE, McCulloch EA. (1971) Mouse myeloma tumor stem cells: a primary cell culture assay. *J. Natl. Cancer Inst.* 46:411-422.

[28] Bruce WR, Van Der Gaag H. (1963) A quantitative assay for the number of murine lymphoma cells capableof proliferation in vivo. *Nature* 199:79-80.

[29] Hamburger AW, Salmon SE (1977) Primary bioassay of human tumor stem cells. *Science* 197:461-463.

[30] Bergsagel DE, Valeriote FA. (1968) Growth characteristics of a mouse plasma cell tumor.*Cancer Res.* 28:2187-2196.

[31] Southam CM, Brunschwig A, (1968) A quantitative studies of autotransplantation of human cancer. *Cancer* 14: 971-978.

[32] Fidler IJ, Kripke ML. (1977) Metastasis results from preexisting variant cells within a malignant tumor. *Science* 197:893-895.

[33] Nowell PC (1986) Mechanisms of tumor progression. *Cancer Res*. 46:2203-2207.

[34] Lapidot T, Sirard C, Vormoor J, Murdoch B, Hoang T, Caceres-Cortes J, Minden M, Paterson B, Caligiuri MA, Dick JE. (1994) A cell initiating human acute myeloid leukaemia after transplantation into SCID mice. *Nature* 367:645-648.

[35] Bonnet D, Dick JE. (1997) Human acute myeloid leukemia is organized as a hierarchy that originates from a primitive hematopoietic cell. *Nat. Med.* 3:730-737.

[36] Marx J (2003) Cancer research. Mutant stem cells may seed cancer. *Science* 301:1308-1310.

[37] Park IK, Qian D, Kiel M, Becker MW, Pihalja M, Weissman IL, Morrison SJ, Clarke MF. (2003) Bmi-1 is required for maintenance of adult self-renewing haematopoietic stem cells. *Nature* 423:302-305.

[38] Lessard J, Sauvageau G. (2003) Bmi-1 determines the proliferative capacity of normal and leukaemic stem cells. *Nature* 423:255-260.

[39] Taipale J, Beachy PA. (2001) The Hedgehog and Wnt signalling pathways in cancer. *Nature* 411:349-354.

[40] Reya T, Clevers H. (2005) Wnt signalling in stem cells and cancer. *Nature* 434:843-350.

[41] Beachy PA, Karhadkar SS, Berman DM (2004) Tissue repair and stem cell renewal in carcinogenesis. *Nature* 432:324-331.

[42] Woodward WA, Chen MS, Behbod F, Rosen JM. (2005) On mammary stem cells. *J. Cell Sci.* 118:3585-3594.

[43] Park IK, Morrison SJ, Clarke MF. (2004) Bmi1, stem cells, and senescence regulation. *J. Clin. Invest.* 113:175-179.

[44] Valk-Lingbeek ME, Bruggeman SW, van Lohuizen M. (2004) Stem cells and cancer; the polycomb connection. *Cell* 118:409-418.

[45] Leung C, Lingbeek M, Shakhova O, Liu J, Tanger E, Saremaslani P, Van Lohuizen M, Marino S. (2004) Bmi1 is essential for cerebellar development and is overexpressed in human medulloblastomas. *Nature* 428:337-341.

[46] Kim JH, Yoon SY, Jeong SH, Kim SY, Moon SK, Joo JH, Lee Y, Choe IS, Kim JW. (2004) Overexpression of Bmi-1 oncoprotein correlates with axillary lymph node metastases in invasive ductal breast cancer. *Breast* 13:383-388.

[47] Behrens J, Lustig B. (2004) The Wnt connection to tumorigenesis. *Int. J. Dev. Biol.* 48: 477-487.

[48] Fuchs SY, Ougolkov AV, Spiegelman VS, Minamoto T. (2005) Oncogenic beta-catenin signaling networks in colorectal cancer. *Cell Cycle* 4:1522-1539.

[49] Cho KH, Baek S, Sung MH. (2006) Wnt pathway mutations selected by optimal beta-catenin signaling for tumorigenesis. *FEBS Lett.* 580:3665-3670.

[50] Hirabayashi Y, Itoh Y, Tabata H, Nakajima K, Akiyama T, Masuyama N, Gotoh Y. (2004) The Wnt/beta-catenin pathway directs neuronal differentiation of cortical neural precursor cells. *Development* 131:2791-2801.

[51] Dorsky RI, Moon RT, Raible DW. (1998) Control of neural crest cell fate by the Wnt signalling pathway. *Nature* 396:370-373.

[52] Lee HY, Kleber M, Hari L, Brault V, Suter U, Taketo MM, Kemler R, Sommer L. (2004) Instructive role of Wnt/beta-catenin in sensory fate specification in neural crest stem cells. *Science* 303:1020-1023.

[53] Kleber M, Lee HY, Wurdak H, Buchstaller J, Riccomagno MM, Ittner LM, Suter U, Epstein DJ, Sommer L. (2005) Neural crest stem cell maintenance by combinatorial Wnt and BMP signaling. *J. Cell Biol.* 169:309-320.

[54] Ingham PW. (1998) Transducing Hedgehog: the story so far. *EMBO J.* 17:3505-3511.

[55] Riobo NA, Lu K, Emerson CP Jr. (2006) Hedgehog Signal Transduction: Signal Integration and Cross Talk In Development and Cancer. *Cell Cycle* 15:1612-1615.

[56] Daya-Grosjean L, Couve-Privat S. (2005) Sonic hedgehog signaling in basal cell carcinomas. *Cancer Lett.* 225:181-192.

[57] Karhadkar SS, Bova GS, Abdallah N, Dhara S, Gardner D, Maitra A, Isaacs JT, Berman DM, Beachy PA. (2004) Hedgehog signalling in prostate regeneration, neoplasia and metastasis. *Nature* 431:707-712.

[58] Stecca B, Ruiz i Altaba A. (2005) Brain as a paradigm of organ growth: Hedgehog-Gli signaling in neural stem cells and brain tumors. *J. Neurobiol.* 64:476-490.

[59] Lees C, Howie S, Sartor RB, Satsangi J. (2005) The hedgehog signalling pathway in the gastrointestinal tract: implications for development, homeostasis, and disease. *Gastroenterology* 129:1696-1710.

[60] Kasper M, Regl G, Frischauf AM, Aberger F. (2006) GLI transcription factors: mediators of oncogenic Hedgehog signalling. *Eur. J. Cancer* 42:437-445.

[61] Androutsellis-Theotokis A, Leker RR, Soldner F, Hoeppner DJ, Ravin R, Poser SW, Rueger MA, Bae SK, Kittappa R, McKay RD. (2006) Notch signalling regulates stem cell numbers in vitro and in vivo. *Nature* 442:823-826.

[62] Radtke F, Wilson A, Mancini SJ, MacDonald HR. (2004) Notch regulation of lymphocyte development and function. *Nat. Immunol.* 5:247-253.

[63] Lasky JL, Wu H. (2005) Notch signaling, brain development, and human disease. *Pediatr. Res.* 57:104R-109R.

[64] Katsube K, Sakamoto K. (2005) Notch in vertebrates--molecular aspects of the signal. *Int. J. Dev. Biol.* 49:369-374.

[65] Luo D, Renault VM, Rando TA. (2005) The regulation of Notch signaling in muscle stem cell activation and postnatal myogenesis. *Semin. Cell Dev. Biol.* 16:612-622.

[66] Suzuki T, Chiba S. (2005) Notch signaling in hematopoietic stem cells. *Int. J. Hematol.* 82: 285-294.

[67] Wilson A, Radtke F. (2006) Multiple functions of Notch signaling in self-renewing organs and cancer. *FEBS Lett.* 580:2860-2868.

[68] Radtke F, Clevers H, Riccio O. (2006) From gut homeostasis to cancer. *Curr. Mol. Med.* 6: 275-289.

[69] Selleck MA, Scherson TY, Bronner-Fraser M. (1993) Origins of neural crest cell diversity. *Dev. Biol.* 159:1-11.

[70] Nakagawara A. (2004) Neural crest development and neuroblastoma: the genetic and biological link. *Prog. Brain Res.* 146:233-242.

[71] Komuro H, Hayashi Y, Kawamura M, Hayashi K, Kaneko Y, Kamoshita S, Hanada R, Yamamoto K, Hongo T, Yamada M, Tsuchida Y. (1993) Mutations of the p53 gene are involved in Ewing's sarcomas but not in neuroblastomas. *Cancer Res.* 53:5284-288.

[72] Brodeur GM. (2003) Neuroblastoma: biological insights into a clinical enigma. *Nat. Rev. Cancer* 3:203-216.

[73] Nowak K, Kerl K, Fehr D, Kramps C, Gessner C, Killmer K, Samans B, Berwanger B, Christiansen H, Lutz W. (2006) BMI1 is a target gene of E2F-1 and is strongly expressed in primary neuroblastomas. *Nucleic Acids Res.* 34:1745-1754.

[74] Blanc E, Goldschneider D, Douc-Rasy S, Benard J, Raguenez G. (2005) Wnt-5a gene expression in malignant human neuroblasts. *Cancer Lett.* 228:117-123.

[75] Blanc E, Roux GL, Benard J, Raguenez G. (2005) Low expression of Wnt-5a gene is associated with high-risk neuroblastoma. *Oncogene* 24:1277-1283.

[76] Pahlman S, Stockhausen MT, Fredlund E, Axelson H (2004) Notch signaling in neuroblastoma. *Semin. Cancer Biol.* 14:365-373.

[77] Axelson H. (2004) The Notch signaling cascade in neuroblastoma: role of the basic helix-loop-helix proteins HASH-1 and HES-1. *Cancer Lett.* 204:171-178.

[78] Goodell MA, Brose K, Paradis G, Conner AS, Mulligan RC. (1996) Isolation and functional properties of murine hematopoietic stem cells that are replicating in vivo. *J. Exp. Med.* 183:1797-1806.

[79] Asakura A, Seale P, Girgis-Gabardo A, Rudnicki MA. (2002) Myogenic specification of side population cells in skeletal muscle. *J. Cell Biol.* 159:123-134.

[80] Welm BE, Tepera SB, Venezia T, Graubert TA, Rosen JM, Goodell MA. (2002) Sca-1(pos) cells in the mouse mammary gland represent an enriched progenitor cell population. *Dev. Biol.* 245:42-56.

[81] Triel C, Vestergaard ME, Bolund L, Jensen TG, Jensen UB. (2004) Side population cells in human and mouse epidermis lack stem cell characteristics. *Exp. Cell Res.* 295: 79-90.

[82] Summer R, Kotton DN, Sun X, Ma B, Fitzsimmons K, Fine A. (2003) Side population cells and Bcrp1 expression in lung. *Am. J. Physiol. Lung Cell Mol. Physiol.* 285:L97-104.

[83] Murayama A, Matsuzaki Y, Kawaguchi A, Shimazaki T, Okano H. (2002) Flow cytometric analysis of neural stem cells in the developing and adult mouse brain. J. *Neurosci. Res.* 69:837-847.

[84] 'Lassalle B, Bastos H, Louis JP, Riou L, Testart J, Dutrillaux B, Fouchet P, Allemand I. (2004) Side Population' cells in adult mouse testis express Bcrp1 gene and are enriched in spermatogonia and germinal stem cells. *Development* 131:479-487.

[85] Hussain SZ, Strom SC, Kirby MR, Burns S, Langemeijer S, Ueda T, Hsieh M, Tisdale JF. (2005) Side population cells derived from adult human liver generate hepatocyte-like cells in vitro. *Dig. Dis. Sci.* 50:1755-1763.

[86] Iwatani H, Ito T, Imai E, Matsuzaki Y, Suzuki A, Yamato M, Okabe M, Hori M. (2004) Hematopoietic and nonhematopoietic potentials of Hoechst(low)/side population cells isolated from adult rat kidney. *Kidney Int.* 65:1604-1614.

[87] Rochon C, Frouin V, Bortoli S, Giraud-Triboult K, Duverger V, Vaigot P, Petat C, Fouchet P, Lassalle B, Alibert O, Gidrol X, Pietu G. (2006) Comparison of gene expression pattern in SP cell populations from four tissues to define common "stemness functions". *Exp. Cell Res.* 312:2074-2082.

[88] Hirschmann-Jax C, Foster AE, Wulf GG, Nuchtern JG, Jax TW, Gobel U, Goodell MA, Brenner MK. (2004) A distinct "side population" of cells with high drug efflux capacity in human tumor cells. *Proc. Natl. Acad. Sci. USA* 101:14228-14233.

[89] Kondo T, Setoguchi T, Taga T. (2004) Persistence of a small subpopulation of cancer stem-like cells in the C6 glioma cell line. *Proc. Natl. Acad. Sci. USA* 101:781-786.

[90] Haraguchi N, Utsunomiya T, Inoue H, Tanaka F, Mimori K, Barnard GF, Mori M. (2006) Characterization of a side population of cancer cells from human gastrointestinal system. *Stem Cells* 24:506-513.

[91] Chiba T, Kita K, Zheng YW, Yokosuka O, Saisho H, Iwama A, Nakauchi H, Taniguchi H. (2006) Side population purified from hepatocellular carcinoma cells harbors cancer stem cell-like properties. *Hepatology* 44:240-251.

[92] Szotek PP, Pieretti-Vanmarcke R, Masiakos PT, Dinulescu DM, Connolly D, Foster R, Dombkowski D, Preffer F, Maclaughlin DT, Donahoe PK. (2006) Ovarian cancer side population defines cells with stem cell-like characteristics and Mullerian Inhibiting Substance responsiveness. *Proc. Natl. Acad. Sci. USA* 103:11154-11159.

[93] Singh SK, Clarke ID, Terasaki M, Bonn VE, Hawkins C, Squire J, Dirks PB. (2003) Identification of a cancer stem cell in human brain tumors. Cancer Res. 63:5821-5828.

[94] Al-Hajj M, Wicha MS, Benito-Hernandez A, Morrison SJ, Clarke MF. (2003) Prospective identification of tumorigenic breast cancer cells. *Proc. Natl. Acad. Sci. USA* 100:3983-3988.

[95] Jacques TS, Relvas JB, Nishimura S, Pytela R, Edwards GM, Streuli CH, ffrench-Constant C. (1998) Neural precursor cell chain migration and division are regulated through different beta1 integrins. *Development* 125:3167-3177.

[96] Dontu G, Abdallah WM, Foley JM, Jackson KW, Clarke MF, Kawamura MJ, Wicha MS. (2003) In vitro propagation and transcriptional profiling of human mammary stem/progenitor cells. *Genes Dev.* 17:1253-1270.

[97] Hemmati HD, Nakano I, Lazareff JA, Masterman-Smith M, Geschwind DH, Bronner-Fraser M, Kornblum HI. (2003) Cancerous stem cells can arise from pediatric brain tumors. *Proc. Natl. Acad. Sci. USA* 100:15178-15183.

[98] Ponti D, Costa A, Zaffaroni N, Pratesi G, Petrangolini G, Coradini D, Pilotti S, Pierotti MA, Daidone MG. (2005) Isolation and in vitro propagation of tumorigenic breast cancer cells with stem/progenitor cell properties. *Cancer Res.* 65:5506-5511.

[99] Ross RA, Spengler BA, Domenech C, Porubcin M, Rettig WJ, Biedler JL. (1995) Human neuroblastoma I-type cells are malignant neural crest stem cells. *Cell Growth Differ.* 6:449-456.

[100] Ross RA, Spengler BA. (2004) The conundrum posed by cellular heterogeneity in analysis of human neuroblastoma. *J. Natl. Cancer Inst.* 96:1192-1193.

[101] Walton JD, Kattan DR, Thomas SK, Spengler BA, Guo HF, Biedler JL, Cheung NK, Ross RA. (2004) Characteristics of stem cells from human neuroblastoma cell lines and in tumors. *Neoplasia* 6:838-845.

[102] Ross RA, Spengler BA. (2006) Human neuroblastoma stem cells. *Semin. Cancer Biol.*

[103] Wulf GG, Wang RY, Kuehnle I, Weidner D, Marini F, Brenner MK, Andreeff M, Goodell MA. (2001) A leukemic stem cell with intrinsic drug efflux capacity in acute myeloid leukemia. *Blood* 98:1166-1173.

[104] Sarkadi B, Ozvegy-Laczka C, Nemet K, Varadi A. (2004) ABCG2 -- a transporter for all seasons. *FEBS Lett.* 567:116-120.

[105] Dean M, Fojo T, Bates S. (2005) Tumour stem cells and drug resistance. *Nat. Rev. Cancer* 5:275-284.

[106] Leslie EM, Deeley RG, Cole SP. (2005) Multidrug resistance proteins: role of P-glycoprotein, MRP1, MRP2, and BCRP (ABCG2) in tissue defense. *Toxicol. Appl. Pharmacol.* 204:216-237.

[107] Szakacs G, Paterson JK, Ludwig JA, Booth-Genthe C, Gottesman MM. (2006) Targeting multidrug resistance in cancer. *Nat. Rev. Drug Discov.* 5:219-234.

[108] Bunting KD. (2002) ABC transporters as phenotypic markers and functional regulators of stem cells. *Stem Cells* 20:11-20.

[109] Zhou S, Schuetz JD, Bunting KD, Colapietro AM, Sampath J, Morris JJ, Lagutina I, Grosveld GC, Osawa M, Nakauchi H, Sorrentino BP. (2001) The ABC transporter Bcrp1/ABCG2 is expressed in a wide variety of stem cells and is a molecular determinant of the side-population phenotype. *Nat. Med.* 7:1028-1034.

[110] Goldstein LJ, Fojo AT, Ueda K, Crist W, Green A, Brodeur G, Pastan I, Gottesman MM. (1990) Expression of the multidrug resistance, MDR1, gene in neuroblastomas. *J. Clin. Oncol.* 8:128-136.

[111] Norris MD, Bordow SB, Marshall GM, Haber PS, Cohn SL, Haber M. (1996) Expression of the gene for multidrug-resistance-associated protein and outcome in patients with neuroblastoma. *N. Engl. J. Med.* 334:231-238.

[112] Peaston AE, Gardaneh M, Franco AV, Hocker JE, Murphy KM, Farnsworth ML, Catchpoole DR, Haber M, Norris MD, Lock RB, Marshall GM. (2001) MRP1 gene expression level regulates the death and differentiation response of neuroblastoma cells. *Br. J. Cancer* 85:1564-1571.

[113] Haber M, Smith J, Bordow SB, Flemming C, Cohn SL, London WB, Marshall GM, Norris MD. (2006) Association of high-level MRP1

expression with poor clinical outcome in a large prospective study of primary neuroblastoma. *J. Clin. Oncol.* 24: 1546-1553.

[114] Lepourcelet M, Chen YN, France DS, Wang H, Crews P, Petersen F, Bruseo C, Wood AW, Shivdasani RA. (2004) Small-molecule antagonists of the oncogenic Tcf/beta-catenin protein complex. *Cancer Cell* 5:91-102.

[115] Luu HH, Zhang R, Haydon RC, Rayburn E, Kang Q, Si W, Park JK, Wang H, Peng Y, Jiang W, He TC. (2004) Wnt/beta-catenin signaling pathway as a novel cancer drug target. *Curr. Cancer Drug Targets* 4:653-671.

[116] Mimeault M, Batra SK. (2006) Recent advances on multiple tumorigenic cascades involved in prostatic cancer progression and targeting therapies. *Carcinogenesis* 27:1-22.

[117] Galmozzi E, Facchetti F, La Porta CA. (2006) Cancer stem cells and therapeutic perspectives. *Curr. Med. Chem.* 13:603-607.

[118] Chen JK, Taipale J, Cooper MK, Beachy PA. (2002) Inhibition of hedgehog signaling by direct binding of cyclopamine to smoothened. *Genes. Dev.* 16:2743–2748.

[119] Berman DM, Karhadkar SS, Hallahan AR, Pritchard JI, Eberhart CG, Watkins DN, Chen JK, Cooper MK, Taipale J, Olson JM, Beachy PA. (2002) Medulloblastoma growth inhibition by hedgehog pathway blockade. *Science* 297:1559-1561.

[120] Romer J, Curran T. (2005) Targeting medulloblastoma: small-molecule inhibitors of the Sonic Hedgehog pathway as potential cancer therapeutics. *Cancer Res.* 65:4975-4978.

[121] Williams JA, Guicherit OM, Zaharian BI, Xu Y, Chai L, Wichterle H, Kon C, Gatchalian C, Porter JA, Rubin LL, Wang FY. (2003) Identification of a small molecule inhibitor of the hedgehog signaling pathway: effects on basal cell carcinoma-like lesions. *Proc. Natl. Acad. Sci. USA* 100:4616-4621.

[122] Curry CL, Reed LL, Golde TE, Miele L, Nickoloff BJ, Foreman KE. (2005) Gamma secretase inhibitor blocks Notch activation and induces apoptosis in Kaposi's sarcoma tumor cells. *Oncogene* 24:6333-6344.

[123] Katoh M, Katoh M. (2006) NUMB is a break of WNT - Notch signaling cycle. *Int. J. Mol. Med.* 18:517-521.

[124] Belpomme D, Gauthier S, Pujade-Lauraine E, Facchini T, Goudier MJ, Krakowski I, Netter-Pinon G, Frenay M, Gousset C, Marie FN, Benmiloud M, Sturtz F. (2000) Verapamil increases the survival of patients with anthracycline-resistant metastatic breast carcinoma. *Ann. Oncol.* 11:1471-1476.

[125] Slater LM, Sweet P, Stupecky M, Gupta S. (1986) Cyclosporin A reverses vincristine and daunorubicin resistance in acute lymphatic leukemia in vitro. *J. Clin. Invest* 77: 1405-1408.

[126] Friedenberg WR, Rue M, Blood EA, Dalton WS, Shustik C, Larson RA, Sonneveld P, Greipp PR. (2006) Phase III study of PSC-833 (valspodar) in combination with vincristine, doxorubicin, and dexamethasone (valspodar/VAD) versus VAD alone in patients with recurring or refractory multiple myeloma (E1A95): a trial of the Eastern Cooperative Oncology Group. *Cancer* 106:830-838.

[127] Minderman H, O'Loughlin KL, Pendyala L, Baer MR. (2004) VX-710 (biricodar) increases drug retention and enhances chemosensitivity in resistant cells overexpressing P-glycoprotein, multidrug resistance protein, and breast cancer resistance protein. *Clin. Cancer Res.* 10:1826-1834.

[128] Sandler A, Gordon M, De Alwis DP, Pouliquen I, Green L, Marder P, Chaudhary A, Fife K, Battiato L, Sweeney C, Jordan C, Burgess M, Slapak CA. (2004) A Phase I trial of a potent P-glycoprotein inhibitor, zosuquidar trihydrochloride (LY335979), administered intravenously in combination with doxorubicin in patients with advanced malignancy. *Clin. Cancer Res.* 10:3265-3272.

[129] Mistry P, Plumb J, Eccles S, Watson S, Dale I, Ryder H, Box G, Charlton P, Templeton D, Bevan PB. (1999) In vivo efficacy of XR9051, a potent modulator of P-glycoprotein mediated multidrug resistance. *Br. J. Cancer* 79:1672-1678.

[130] Mistry P, Stewart AJ, Dangerfield W, Okiji S, Liddle C, Bootle D, Plumb JA, Templeton D, Charlton P. (2001) In vitro and in vivo reversal of P-glycoprotein-mediated multidrug resistance by a novel potent modulator, XR9576. *Cancer Res.* 61: 749-758.

[131] de Bruin M, Miyake K, Litman T, Robey R, Bates SE. (1999) Reversal of resistance by GF120918 in cell lines expressing the ABC half-transporter, MXR. *Cancer Lett.* 146: 117-126.

[132] Robey RW, Steadman K, Polgar O, Morisaki K, Blayney M, Mistry P, Bates SE. (2004) Pheophorbide a is a specific probe for ABCG2 function and inhibition. *Cancer Res.* 64: 1242-1246.

[133] Brooks TA, Minderman H, O'Loughlin KL, Pera P, Ojima I, Baer MR, Bernacki RJ. (2003) Taxane-based reversal agents modulate drug resistance mediated by P-glycoprotein, multidrug resistance protein, and breast cancer resistance protein. *Mol. Cancer Ther.* 2:1195-1205.

[134] Patrawala L, Calhoun T, Schneider-Broussard R, Zhou J, Claypool K, Tang DG. (2005) Side population is enriched in tumorigenic, stem-like cancer cells, whereas ABCG2+ and ABCG2- cancer cells are similarly tumorigenic. *Cancer Res.* 65:6207-6219.

[135] Tsimberidou AM, Giles FJ, Estey E, O'Brien S, Keating MJ, Kantarjian HM. (2006) The role of gemtuzumab ozogamicin in acute leukaemia therapy. *Br. J. Haematol.* 132: 398-409.

[136] Ponzoni M, Bocca P, Chiesa V, Decensi A, Pistoia V, Raffaghello L, Rozzo C, Montaldo PG. (1995) Differential effects of N-(4-hydroxyphenyl)retinamide and retinoic acid on neuroblastoma cells: apoptosis versus differentiation. *Cancer Res.* 55: 853-861.

[137] Kim CJ, Kim HO, Choe YJ, Lee YA, Kim CW. (1995) Bcl-2 expression in neuroblastoma is differentially regulated by differentiation inducers. *Anticancer Res.* 15: 1997-2000.

[138] Niizuma H, Nakamura Y, Ozaki T, Nakanishi H, Ohira M, Isogai E, Kageyama H, Imaizumi M, Nakagawara A. (2006) Bcl-2 is a key regulator for the retinoic acid-induced apoptotic cell death in neuroblastoma. *Oncogene* 25:5046-55.

[139] Pahlman S, Ruusala AI, Abrahamsson L, Mattsson ME, Esscher T. (1984) Retinoic acid-induced differentiation of cultured human neuroblastoma cells: a comparison with phorbolester-induced differentiation. *Cell Differ.* 14:135-144.

[140] Jensen LM, Zhang Y, Shooter EM. (1992) Steady-state polypeptide modulations associated with nerve growth factor (NGF)-induced terminal differentiation and NGF deprivation-induced apoptosis in human neuroblastoma cells. *J. Biol. Chem.* 267: 19325-19333.

[141] Kuner P, Hertel C. (1998) NGF induces apoptosis in a human neuroblastoma cell line expressing the neurotrophin receptor p75NTR. *J. Neurosci. Res.* 54:465-474.

[142] Jogi A, Ora I, Nilsson H, Lindeheim A, Makino Y, Poellinger L, Axelson H, Pahlman S. (2002) Hypoxia alters gene expression in human neuroblastoma cells toward an immature and neural crest-like phenotype. *Proc. Natl. Acad. Sci. USA* 99:7021-7026.

[143] Jogi A, Vallon-Christersson J, Holmquist L, Axelson H, Borg A, Pahlman S. (2004) Human neuroblastoma cells exposed to hypoxia: induction of genes associated with growth, survival, and aggressive behavior. *Exp. Cell Res.* 295:469-487.

[144] Axelson H, Fredlund E, Ovenberger M, Landberg G, Pahlman S. (2005) Hypoxia-induced dedifferentiation of tumor cells--a mechanism behind heterogeneity and aggressiveness of solid tumors. *Semin. Cell Dev. Biol.* 16:554-563.

[145] Edsjo A, Holmquist L, Pahlman S. (2006) Neuroblastoma as an experimental model for neuronal differentiation and hypoxia-induced tumor cell dedifferentiation. *Semin. Cancer Biol.* In press.

[146] Dean M (1998) Cancer as a complex developmental disorder--nineteenth Cornelius P. Rhoads Memorial Award Lecture. *Cancer Res.* 58:5633-5636.

[147] Yamashita YM, Fuller MT, Jones DL. (2005) Signaling in stem cell niches: lessons from the Drosophila germline. *J. Cell Sci.* 118:665-672.

[148] Chepko G, Slack R, Carbott D, Khan S, Steadman L, Dickson RB. (2005) Differential alteration of stem and other cell populations in ducts and lobules of TGFalpha and c-Myc transgenic mouse mammary epithelium. *Tissue Cell* 37:393-412.

[149] Polyak K, Hu M. (2005) Do myoepithelial cells hold the key for breast tumor progression? *J. Mammary Gland Biol. Neoplasia* 10:231-247.

[150] Ambros IM, Attarbaschi A, Rumpler S, Luegmayr A, Turkof E, Gadner H, Ambros PF. (2001) Neuroblastoma cells provoke Schwann cell proliferation in vitro. *Med. Pediatr Oncol.* 36:163-168.

[151] Liu S, Tian Y, Chlenski A, Yang Q, Zage P, Salwen HR, Crawford SE, Cohn SL. (2005) Cross-talk between Schwann cells and neuroblasts influences the biology of neuroblastoma xenografts. *Am. J. Pathol.* 166:891-900.

[152] Mora J, Cheung NK, Juan G, Illei P, Cheung I, Akram M, Chi S, Ladanyi M, Cordon-Cardo C, Gerald WL. (2001) Neuroblastic and Schwannian stromal cells of neuroblastoma are derived from a tumoral progenitor cell. *Cancer Res.* 61:6892-6898.

[153] Coco S, Defferrari R, Scaruffi P, Cavazzana A, Di Cristofano C, Longo L, Mazzocco K, Perri P, Gambini C, Moretti S, Bonassi S, Tonini GP. (2005) Genome analysis and gene expression profiling of neuroblastoma and ganglioneuroblastoma reveal differences between neuroblastic and Schwannian stromal cells. *J. Pathol.* 207:346-357.

[154] Ambros IM, Ambros PF. (1995) Schwann cells in neuroblastoma. *Eur. J. Cancer* 31A: 429-34.

[155] Kwiatkowski JL, Rutkowski JL, Yamashiro DJ, Tennekoon GI, Brodeur GM. (1998) Schwann cell-conditioned medium promotes neuroblastoma survival and differentiation. *Cancer Res.* 58:4602-4606.

[156] Huang D, Rutkowski JL, Brodeur GM, Chou PM, Kwiatkowski JL, Babbo A, Cohn SL. (2000) Schwann cell-conditioned medium inhibits angiogenesis. *Cancer Res.* 60: 5966-5971.

[157] Chlenski A, Liu S, Crawford SE, Volpert OV, DeVries GH, Evangelista A, Yang Q, Salwen HR, Farrer R, Bray J, Cohn SL. (2002) SPARC is a key Schwannian-derived inhibitor controlling neuroblastoma tumor angiogenesis. *Cancer Res.* 62:7357-7363.

[158] Grayson WL, Zhao F, Izadpanah R, Bunnell B, Ma T. (2006) Effects of hypoxia on human mesenchymal stem cell expansion and plasticity in 3D constructs. *J. Cell Physiol.* 207: 331-339.

[159] Yang Z, Levison SW. (2006) Hypoxia/ischemia expands the regenerative capacity of progenitors in the perinatal subventricular zone. *Neuroscience* 139:555-564.

[160] Boccaccio C, Comoglio PM. (2006) Invasive growth: a MET-driven genetic programme for cancer and stem cells. *Nat. Rev. Cancer* 6:637-645.

In: Neuroblastoma Research Trends
Editors: L. H. Andre and N. E. Roux
ISBN: 978-1-60456-790-8

Chapter II

Perspectives of Proteomics Investigations of Neuroblastoma Chemoresistance

Annamaria D'Alessandro[1,2,3], Valeria Marzano[1,2,3], Simona D'Aguanno[1,2,3], Luisa Pieroni[1,4,5], Sergio Bernardini[1,2,3], Giorgio Federici[1,2,3] and Andrea Urbani[1,4,5 2]

1. Children's Hospital "Bambino Gesu' " – IRCCS, Rome, Italy
2. Department of Internal Medicine, University of Rome "Tor Vergata", Rome, Italy
3. Department of Laboratory' Medicine, University Hospital of Rome "Tor Vergata", Rome, Italy
4. Centro Studi sull'Invecchiamento (Ce.S.I.), University Foundation "G.D'Annunzio", Chieti, Italy
5. Department of Biomedical Science, University of Chieti and Pescara "G. D'Annunzio",Chieti, Italy

[2] Corresponding author: Prof. Andrea Urbani, University of Chieti and Pescara "G. D'Annunzio", Department of Biomedical Science, Via Colle dell'Ara (CeSI), 66013-CHIETI, ITALY; e-mail: a.urbani@unich.it; tel: +39-0871-541580; FAX: +39-0871-541598.

Abstract

Neuroblastoma, the third most common paediatric solid tumors after leukaemiae and brain neoplasiae, with an incidence of approximately 1.3 child out of 100.000, is responsible of 15% of all childhood cancer death.

The acquisition of multidrug resistance upon treatment with anticancer drugs is a common feature of highly malignant Neuroblastoma. The identification of marker proteins involved in chemo-resistance might significantly help in the prognosis of this neoplasia by individualising the drug treatment .

Proteomics investigation might represent a powerful holistic scientific approach in order to possibly characterised the molecular hallmarks of Neuroblastoma chemoresistance. Combining high-resolution protein separations with mass spectrometry protein identification, proteomics allows to explore the molecular mechanisms of cancer chemoresistance in a data driven experimental design, therefore enabling the construction of novel hypothesis not necessarily linked to a define researcher theory.

In the following we review the current state of the art in the proteomics investigations devoted to the characterisation of Neuroblastoma drug resistance.

Keywords: *Proteomics, Neuroblastoma, Chemoresistance, Pediatry, Cancer.*

Introduction

Neuroblastoma is the most common extracranial tumor of childhood and the most common cancer diagnosed during infancy, at a median age of 18 months (Landis S.H. et al., 1999). The incidence of this tumor is fairly uniform throughout the world; the aetiology of neuroblastoma is still not clear, but it seems unlikely that environmental exposure has a significant role (Kushner B.H. et al., 1986). This neoplasia is characterized by a heterogeneous clinical behaviour, which have been used for the classification and prognosis of the disease.

Mainly the classification divides Neuroblastoma class of tumors in unfavourable and favourable subtypes, depending on the genetic changes occurred. A subset of patient can inherit a genetic predisposition to neuroblastoma, but mostly somatic gene changes have been shown to be correlated to different tumor subtypes. Usually a favourable prognosis is associated to near triploid karyotypes with whole chromosome gains, rare structural chromosomes rearrangements and high expression of the TrkA neurotrophin receptor. On the contrary unfavourable tumors are characterized by chromosome structural changes (i.e. deletion, or umbalanced gain of a chromosome copy), amplification of the MYCN protooncogene and expression of the TrkB neurotrophin receptor and its ligand (Brodeur G.M., 2003).

A heterogeneous histology is also characteristic for this tumor which derived from developing neural crest, an organ rich of multipotent cells, that give rise multiple cell phenotypes. The International Neuroblastoma Pathological Classification (INPC) has also established histological favourable and unfavourable types that, in combination with the genetic markers can be prognostic for the tumor (Shimada H. et al., 1999).

Distinct Cell Type of Neuroblastoma

To proceed with research studies aimed to better understand aetiology progression and possible therapy for NB, the availability of a cellular model resembling tumor heterogeneity is of primary importance. In the last 30 -years course of studies on the growth, differentiation and malignant properties of Neuroblastoma more then 25 different parental cells lines have been examined and among all the cell lines and clones studied three distinct cellular phenotypes have been identified:

- N type, neuroblastic cells that resembles a sympathoadrenal precursor cell in culture, express biochemical markers (enzymes and cell surface receptors) typical of developing neuroblasts, and are tumorigenic;
- S-type, non-neuronal substrate adherent cells representing the glial /melanoblastic precursor, non expressing neuronal markers proteins and non tumorigenic;
- I-type, first described as a cell with intermediate phenotype between N and S subtypes more recently defined as stem cell precursor of the first two types, expressing both N and S cell marker proteins (Ross R.A. et al., 2003).

These three cell types have been recently demonstrated to occur in human NB tumors, by bone marrow aspiration (Valent A. et al., 1999) using laser capture microdissection (Mora J. et al., 2001) and by immunocitochemistry (Ross R.A. et al., 2003) demonstrating that human neuroblastoma cells variants are not an in vitro artifact but are representative of the tumor in vivo.

Cancer Chemoresistance

A common feature of highly malignant neuroblastoma is the acquisition of multidrug resistance (Keshelava N. et al., 1998). Despite the intensive multimodal therapies and the recent advances in combined chemotherapy, the poor clinical outcome and low response to conventional therapy of Neuroblastoma, due to drug resistance in patients with advanced stage, limit efficacy of the effective chemotherapy (Lange B. et al., 2003).

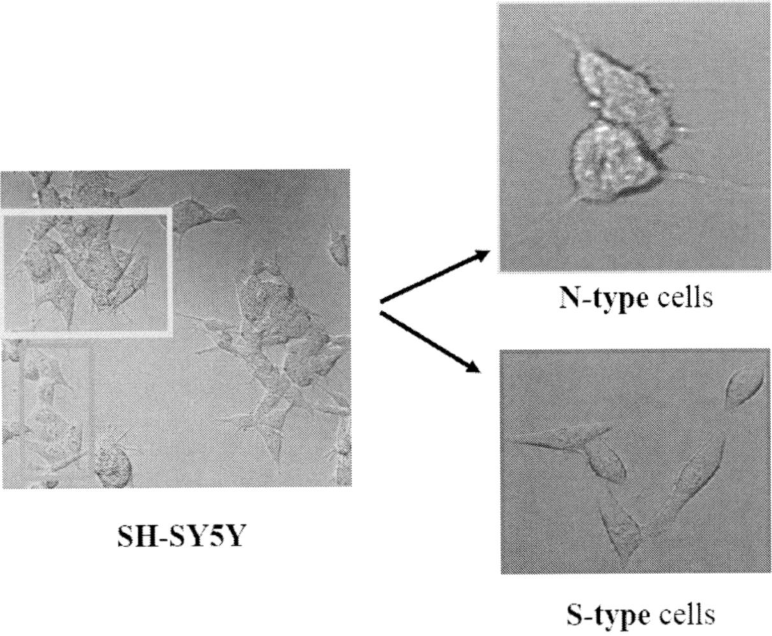

Figure 1. Cytology of Neuroblastoma human cell line : Confocal images of heterogeneous Neuroblastoma human cell line (SH-SY5Y) and sorted subpopulations N-type and S-type.

Table 1. Drug Resistance Mechanisms

Pharmacologic events:	Insufficient drug dose Improper infusion rate Inadequate route of delivery Drug metabolism	References (Castel V., 2001) (Erdlenbruch E., 2001) (Donelli M.G., 1992) (Rivory L.P., 2002)
Cellular events:	Alteration in drug transport systems Modification in drug activation or detoxification Alteration in drug targets Enhanced repair of drug-caused damage Alteration in drug-induced apoptosis Change in signaling pathways	(Juliano R.L., 1976) (Puchalski R.B., 1990) (Kubo T., 1995) (Chaney S.G., 1996) (Wyllie A.H., 1997) (Yu D., 1998)

Neoplastic cells, in fact, can developed an intrinsic (permanent resistance caused by genetic alterations) or an acquired resistance of the cells that, initially are highly responsive to anticancer therapy, but become resistant during the course of the disease.

Multiple cellular mechanism have been identified to contribute to the drug resistance phenotype of cells treated with compounds used in many chemotherapeutic protocols (Table 3). In addition, pharmacologic factors, such as inadequate dosing or route of delivery, may play a role in clinical resistance of tumours (Table 1), (Broker L.E. et al., 2004).

Alterations in drug transport system, that cause a reduced intracellular accumulation of drugs, is one of the most common mechanism of Multi Drug Resistance (MDR). It is caused by enhanced drug efflux or also result from a decreased uptake of the cytotoxic agent caused by defect in the import system (i.e. methotrexate resistance) (Gorlick R. et al., 1997). Many transporter proteins are involved in MDR, such as P-glycoprotein (P-gp) (Juliano R.L. et al., 1976), MDR-associated proteins (MRPs) (Cole S.P. et al., 1992), the transporter associated with antigen presentation (TAP) (Izquierdo M.A. et al., 1996) and others specific for different neoplasiae.

These proteins are able to remove cytotoxic drugs from the cells and can move across cellular membranes against a concentration gradient, by using energy derived from ATP hydrolysis. The best characterized drug exporter is the P-glycoprotein; the substrate list of P-gp contains a wide spectrum of chemotherapeutic drugs, including Vinca alkaloids, Taxanes, Anthracyclines and Epipodophyllotoxins (Litman T. et al., 2001).

An important pathway that leads to inactivation of anticancer drugs is the glutathione/glutathione-S-transferase (GSH/GST) system that conjugates electrophilic metabolites, such as alkylating agents, cisplatin and doxorubicin, with the intracellular antioxidant GSH (Puchalski R.B. et al., 1990). A lot of drugs, such as Methotrexate, to perform their cytotoxic function, needs to be modified, by polyglutamylation, essential mechanism for the retention of the drug in the cells. Polyglutamylated methotrexate is not recognized by export proteins such as MRP (Zeng H. et al., 2001) and can accumulate inside the cell (Gorlick R. et al., 1999).

Alteration in the cellular targets of chemotherapeutic drugs may disturb effective drug-target interaction and thus lead to impaired drug response; defect in topoisomerases, thymidylate synthase, β-tubulin and dihydrofolate reductase, may render tumour cells resistant to drugs that target these proteins. Topoisomerase I and II, enzymes involved in the DNA replication, transcription, chromosome segregation and DNA recombination, are specific targets for the topoisomerase inhibitors (irinotecan, topotecan and etoposide) and alterations of these enzymes lead to resistance against topoisomerase inhibitors in vitro (Kubo T. et al., 1995). In addiction binding of Paclitaxel to β-tubulin (a microtubule-disrupting agent) induces polymerization and bundling of microtubules, which leads to cell-cycle arrest and subsequent cell death (Schiff P.B. et al., 1979).

To preserve genome integrity, cells use a complex machinery to repair the accidental lesions that occur in DNA; these repair damage processes are induced by the action of anticancer drugs and result increased in cells that shown resistance (Chaney S.G. et al., 1996). Four pathways, summarized in Table 2, are involved in the repair of DNA damage induced by anticancer drugs.

Deregulation of apoptotic pathway favors carcinogenesis by providing tumours cells with a survival advantage (Wyllie A.H., 1997). In addiction, because many anticancer agents exert their effect at least through activation of the apoptotic cascade (Fisher D.E., 1994), alteration in apoptosis can lead to a wide-spectrum of drug resistance intracellular target such as p53 (Smith M.L. et al., 2002), Bcl-2 family members (Reed J.C. et al., 1996), c-myc (Nasi S. et al., 2001) and inhibitors of apoptosis proteins (LaCasse E.C. et al., 1998).

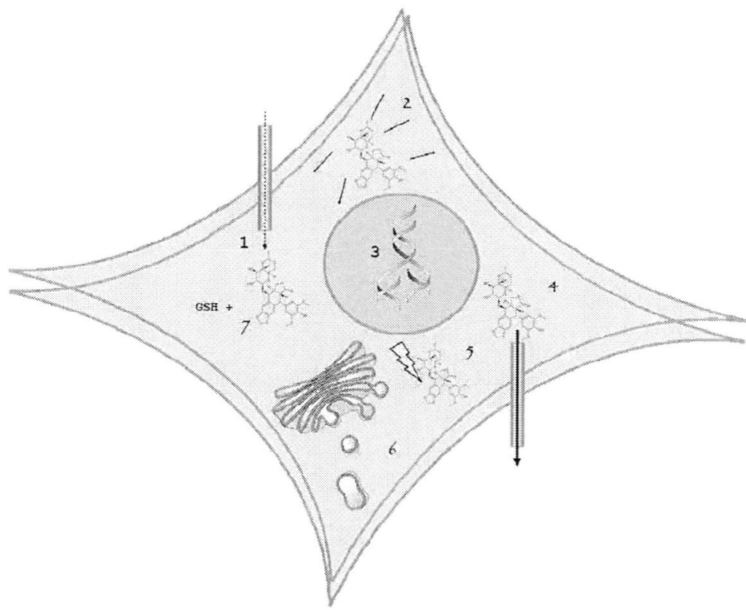

Figure 2. Schematic representation of resistance mechanism : 1) Reduced entry of the drug (i.e. reduced permeability of membrane); 2) Reduced activation of the drug; 3) Promotion of repairing processes of DNA (i.e. ↑ DNA polymerase); 4) Increased ejection of drugs (altered expression of MRPs and P-gp); 5) Increased inactivation of the drug (i.e. ↑ aldehyde dehydrogenase); 6) Altered intracellular distribution of the drug (i.e. toward lysosome); 7) Increase of drug's intracellular link (i.e. GSH).

Cellular processes such as cell proliferation and differentiation are controlled by various signal transduction pathways; the development of biologic response modifiers, which target abnormal signalling pathway in tumours, has led to the recognition of alternative resistance mechanism that stem from alterations in signalling pathways. For example Her-2,a member of the erbB receptor can cause enhanced DNA repair, defective cell-cycle checkpoints and altered apoptoic responses, result in resistance against DNA-damaging agents and antimitotic drugs in vitro (Pietras R.J. et al., 1994).

New therapeutic strategies are therefore needed, including the promising approach represented by specific targeting of drugs, enlucidated by a deep investigation on the neuroblastoma cells' proteome.

Table 2. DNA Repair Mechanisms in Drug Resistance

Repair Mechanism	Drugs involved
Base excision repair	Alkylating agents (Hansen W.K., 2000)
Nucleotide excision repair	Platinum compounds (Furuta T., 2002)
Mismatch repair	/
O^6-alkylguanine DNA alkyltransferase	Nitrosurea-derivatives (Ishiguro K., 2005)

Table 3. Cellular Mechanisms of Resistance against Chemotherapeutic Drugs

Cisplatin	MRPs, Inactivation by Glutathione, Enhanced DNA Repair, Altered Apoptotic Response
Irinotecan	P-gp, Mutation in Topoisomerase I, Degradation of Topoisomerase I-DNA complexes
Paclitaxel	P-gp, β-tubulin Mutations, Altered Apoptotic Response
Methotrexate	MRPs, Decreased Polyglutamylation, Increased Levels of Dihydrofolate Reductase
Doxorubicin	P-gp, MRPs, Mutation in Topoisomerase II, Enhanced DNA Repair, Altered Apoptotic Response

Cell Line Variants as in Vitro Model

As it will be discussed later on in this review, one of the major problem to treat Neuroblastoma at the moment is its ability to develop a resistance to most of chemotherapeutic agent used so far. Therefore, in order to extend the potential results to what occur in the patient, the investigations of drug resistance response and interaction should be pursued with all the cultured neuroblastoma cell variants.

Among all the cell lines already characterized to investigate Neuroblastoma one of the most commonly used is the SH-SY5Y. Those cells are derived from a human neuroblastoma metastasis in bone marrow and are a thrice cloned subline of the neuroblastoma cell line SK-N-SH which was established in 1970 from a metastatic bone tumor. The cells grow as clusters of neuroblastic cells with multiple, short, fine cell processes (neuritis).

The identification of marker proteins involved in chemoresistance mechanisms following an un-bias data driven molecular approach combined differential analysis and protein characterisation by mass spectrometry (MS) will be the focus of this review.

For this kind of studies several cell lines can be employed (i.e. SK-N-SH, IMR32, BE(2)C, N1E-115, etc.) nevertheless the protein content of SH-SY5Y is the most widely characherized so far :

High resolution map of the mitochondrial proteome has been generated by Scheffler N.K. et al. (2001), which produced in those cells a cybrid model for neurodegenerative disorders (Scheffler N.K. et al., 2001);

A profiling of the cell surface proteome of different tumor cell lines including SH-SY5Y, useful to identify novel targets for diagnostic and therapeutic for lots of disease, is available since 2003 (Shin B.K. et al., 2003);

Changes of protein and phosphoroteins profile in SH-SY5Y under oxidative stress (Nakamura M. et al., 2006);

A first proteomic investigation in the field of Neuroblastoma developing drug resistance was pursued to characterize an etoposide chemo-resistant SH-SY5Y derived cloned (Urbani A. et al., 2005).

Human Neuroblastoma Characterization by Proteomic Approach

The aim of a proteomics investigation is to investigate the protein repertoire system biology rather than the role of a single protein. Such a vision considers distinct proteins in their roles as part of a larger system or network. (Liebler D.C., 2002). Different analytical strategies can be followed to achieve the direct analysis and a comprehensive characterization of thousands of proteins (changes in expression, de novo synthesis, new protein isoforms, post-translational modifications, etc) (Figeys D., 2003; Link A.J. et al., 1999; Mann M. et al., 2003): among these the combination of high-resolution two-dimensional electrophoresis (2-DE) and mass spectrometry are the most frequently used.

In the recent years proteome analysis is becoming a key tool in possible new biomarkers discovery, in studying the several cascades involved in the different biological responces, in describing patient serum profiling or in understanding multidrug resistence (MDR) upon treatment with anticancer drugs. An increasing number of studies have been conducted using neuroblastoma as model.

Sitek B. et al. (2005) tried to gain deeper insights into TrkA and TrkB signaling pathways, two biologically active receptors for the neurotrophins involved in growth, survival, and differentiation of normal sympathetic neurons, using the human neuroblastoma SH-SY5Y cell line stably transfected with the TrkA or TrkB cDNA as model system. They used the difference gel electrophoresis (DIGE) system together with MALDI-peptide mass fingerprint (PMF)-MS analysis to identify differences in protein expression. Functional assignment revealed that the majority of these proteins are involved in organization and maintenance of cellular structures. A systematic study for differential expression of signaling proteins (SP) in undifferentiated vs. differentiated cell lineages were performed by Oh J.E. et al. (2005). The N1E-115 cell line was cultivated and an aliquot was differentiated with dimethylsulfoxide (DMSO). Cell lysates were prepared, run on two-dimensional gel electrophoresis (2-DE) followed by MALDI-TOF-TOF identification of proteins and maps of identified SPs were generated. Switching-on/off of several individual SPs from different signaling cascades have been detected during the differentiation. However futher investigations are necessary to understand these process.

Even if the resolving power of 2DE has been improved by the use of more sensitive techniques of protein detection, to increase the likelihood of visualize the low-abundance gene products, complex biological mixtures need to be divided into simpler fractions prior to the proteomic analysis by separating the total protein content into cytosolic, mitochondrial, nuclei and membrane fractions. Scheffler N.K. et al. (2001) obtained mitochondrial fractions by multiple-step percoll/metrizamide gradient . The absence of many membrane-associated proteins known to be associated with these organelles and the limited number of total protein observed in the 2DE gel colloidal coomassie blue maps suggest that the majority of mitochondrial proteins are not being detected under these separation and staining conditions. Fountoulakis M. et al. (2003) obtained one of the larghest organelle databases starting from mitochondrial fraction of the neuroblastoma cell line IMR-32. Protein were resolved by 2DE and stained by coomassie blue. The database comprises 185 different gene products, resulting from the MALDI-MS analysis of approximately 600 spots. The most frequently detected species are heat shock proteins and house-keeping enzymes.

In order to identify novel biomarkers Escobar M.A. et al. (2005) focused their attention on nuclear extracts from three different human NB cell lines SK-N-AS, SK-N-DZ, and SK-N-FI. Proteins were analyzed for differential expression by 2-DE and polypeptides of interest were subsequently identified by liquid chromatography–linked tandem mass spectrometry (LC-MS/MS). They described 20 different proteins, in prelevance oncoproteins, many of which have prior associations with NB and cancer in general. In particular they chose a panel of 3 proteins (SET, grp94, and stathmin) as a potential test for NB detection for future work to validate these proteins as markers in NB by testing other NB cell lines and tissues as well as nonmalignant cells and tissues.

Another cellular compartment of substantial interest is the surface membrane. Comprehensive profiling of proteins expressed on the cell surface could provide a better understanding of the manner in which the cell surface proteome is regulated and how it responds to a variety of intracellular and extracellular signals. Shin B.K. et al. (2003) implemented a biotinylation-based proteome strategy in order to obtain membrane proteins enrichment. Membrane proteins were derivatized with biotin on the surface of intact SH-SY5Y cells. Solubilized biotinylated membrane proteins were purified by avidin column, separated by 2-DE, detected by silver staining and identified by MALDI-TOF-MS or by nanoLC-MS/MS. They identified both glucose-regulated proteins and heat-shock proteins as relatively highly abundant proteins on the cell surface.

Affinity cromatography coupled to mass spectrometry analysis could be a useful tool in investigating the role of proteins like receptors. For example Colabufo N.A. et al. (2006) synthesized a compound with high affinity for the σ_2 receptor to purify by chromatography possible receptor interactors.

Sigma (σ) receptors are classified in σ_1 and σ_2 subtypes and are localized in different tissues, including the central (CNS) and peripheral nervous systems. In the CNS, these receptors are involved in the modulation of neurotransmitter release, in memory and cognitive processes, and in locomotor activity, whereas their role in the peripheral nervous system and their signal transduction have to be clarified. Moreover, σ_1 and σ_2 receptor protein expression in normal tissues is lower than that in the corresponding tumor tissues. In human SK-N-SH neuroblastoma cell line the σ_2 receptors were overexpressed, whereas the σ_1 receptors were found in low affinity state so that they used the human SK-N-SH neuroblastoma as specific in vitro model to perform their experiment.

They characterized the SDS-PAGE gel electrophoresis stained bands by MALDI-MS and LC-MS/MS analysis. The six eluted proteins were identified as human histone proteins. These results disclosed a dual hypothesis about the σ_2 receptor, that it is formed by histones or that the σ_2 ligands also bind histone proteins.

A first attempt to characterize polypeptides repertoire secreted in the media by neuroblastoma cells has been done by Sandoval J.A., Hoelz D.J. et al. (2006). They resolved the secreted proteins by 2-DE gel electrophoresis and LC-MS/MS they identified 5 polypeptides that were secreted or shed by NB. Ubiquitin, b2-microglobulin, insulin-like growth factor binding protein–2, superoxide dismutase (copper and zinc), and heat shock cognate 70-kd proteins were secreted from NB cells, as compared with control media. Elevated levels of these proteins have been described in serum/tissues under intracellular stress and malignancies, including NB. The proteins may reveal additional tumor markers and possibly allow the employment in the diagnosis and treatment of NB. Detection of these proteins in serum of children with NB vs controls using the same approach is currently in progress by the same outhors.

Drug Response Investigations

Resistance to anti-neoplastic drugs is a major clinical problem and the proteomic approach could provide a useful tool in order to discover the mechanism underlying and overcome this trouble.

The aim of our initial study of (Urbani A. et al., 2005) was to determine potential markers of etoposide (a topoisomerase inhibitors extensively used in the treatment of many types of cancer and the most common drug adopted in neuroblastoma chemotherapeutic protocols) resistance in human neuroblastoma cell lines SH-SY5Y. The authors report on a proteomic investigation carried out to map the differential protein expression levels during the exposure of neuroblastoma cell line SH-SY5Y to etoposide. A comparison among parental chemosensitive cell line, parental cell line treated with 1μM etoposide for 10 hours and etoposide-resistant clone cultured with the same concentration of the topoisomerase inhibitor were analyzed by 2-DE and the differentially expressed proteins were identified by MALDI-TOF analysis. In the etoposide exposed SH-SY5Y cell line three protein altered their expression levels: FK506-binding protein 4, cyclophilin A and keratin 9. The first two polypeptides (immunophilines) might protect the cell either acting directly as chaperones towards protein damaged by etoposide or indirectly inducing the over-expression of Pgp. Keratin 9, as all the intermediate filaments, plays a role in dynamic remodelling of cell during development of neoplastic phenotype, execution of apoptosis and maintaining cell integrity. The proteins involved in the establishment of the etoposide resistance are peroxiredoxin1, β-galactoside soluble lectin binding protein, vimentin, Hsp27, hnRNP K, dUTP pyrophosphatase. In particular Hsp27 has the function to augment the cellular survival in stress condition via its chaperone-activity and to modulate the redox state of the cell via the increase of the intracellular abundance of glutathione. This ability of Hsp27 to determine higher levels of glutathione may represent a key point for the study of chemoresistance; in fact it has been established that glutathione is involved in the onset of etoposide resistance in SH-SY5Y cells (Bernardini S. et al., 2002).

Nakamura M. et al. (2006) examined overall protein alteration, including phosphorylation, in the SH-SY5Y cell line under oxidative stress induced by the dopaminergic neurotoxin 6-hydroxydopamine (6-OHDA). The experiments were performed by 2-DE and sequential gel staining with SYPRO Ruby and a novel fluorescent phosphosensor, Pro-Q Diamond Phosphoprotein stain for the detection of phosphorylated forms of protein. For mass spectrometric identification, the authors used a MALDI-TOF MS and a MALDI-QIT-TOF MS/MS instruments. After exposure to 6-OHDA several protein were identified as oxidative stress-responsive elements: elongation factor 2, heat shock cognate 71 kDa protein, lamin A/C, hnRNP H3 and TCP-1, glutathione S-transferase pi. Moreover the phosphorylation state of EF2, lamin A/C, hnRNP H3 and TCP-1 were altered in SH-SY5Y after the treatment. This change in the quantity and status of phosporylation of the identified protein may be an adaptive stress response in order to protects neuronal cells from oxidative stress.

To elucidate the molecular mechanism underlying the oxidative stress-mediated cell-degeneration Ishii T. et al (2005) analyzed the protein carbonylation on SH-SY5Y cells after treatment with an endogenous inducer of ROS production, the 15-deoxy-$\Delta^{12,14}$-prostaglandin J_2 (15d-PGJ_2). After treatment with this compound, biotin-LC-hydrazide was employed to detect protein-bound carbonyls. One-dimensional and two-dimensional electrophoresis were performed and the analysis with MALDI-TOF MS allowed the identification of glutathione-S-transferase P1 and the 19S regulatory cap, S6 ATPase, of the 26S Proteasome as a molecular target of protein oxidation under conditions of electrophile-induced oxidative stress.

All this proteomic studies agree with literature data asserting that some classes of the glutathione-S-transferase might be involved in anticancer-drug-resistance.

Heat shock protein 90 is an interesting anticancer drug target because of its function which is to protect various cellular protein involved in signaling, growth control and survival. Zhang M.H. et al. (2006) identify novel client proteins of Hsp90 and elucidate Hsp90 function through its inhibition by geldanamycin (an agent that exhibits potent antitumor activity). This drug inhibits ATPase activity of Hsp90 by specifically binding to its ATP-binding site and promoting proteolytic degradation of client proteins of Hsp90. Extracts from control and geldanamycin-treated SK-N-SH cells were analyzed by 2-DE and the five polypeptides down-regulated in the treated cells were identified by MALDI-TOF MS. Among these five proteins the authors choose vimentin to test the possibility that this intermediate filament could be a novel Hsp90 target and this result implies that geldanamycin can act as anticancer drug and as an effective chemotherapeutic agent against human neuroblastoma cells promoting the release of vimentin from the Hsp90 complex. This mechanism led to the caspase-dependent vimentin cleavage, which increased sensitivity of the cell to apoptosis-inducing stimuli.

The involvement of one intermediate filament (vimentin) in the foregoing studies points to the importance of the cytoskeletal proteins and their alterated expressions in the onset of cellular resistance to chemotherapeutic agents. Among the several antineoplastic drugs used in neuroblastoma chemotherapeutic protocols, antimicrotubule agents such as paclitaxel, vincristine and vinblastine are extensively used. However resistance to these agents represents the major limit of the antimitotic therapies and the development of drug resistance has been associated with alterations in the drug target or differential expression of tubulin isotypes that confers altered sensitivity to antimicrotubule agents. In a recent study Verrillis N.M. et al. (2006) identified a different molecular mechanism of resistance to anticancer agents that target tubulin: the loss of wild-type γ-actin mediates the failure of the therapy. Proteins of the cytoskeleton from CCRF-CEM cells (a human T-cell acute lymphoblastic leukaemia cell line) and sublines that are resistant to vinblastine or desoxyepothilone B were analyzed for differential expression by 2-DE and the different γ-actin isoforms of the resistant cell lines were identified with MALDI-TOF mass spectrometry. The subsequent ESI-TOF MS/MS revealed the presence of amino acid substitution in the mutant polypeptides of interest that causes the loss of sensitivity toward the anticancer treatment. Trasfecting human neuroblastoma SH-EP cells with siRNA in order to eliminate wt- γ-actin expression suggested the possibility that the drug resistance phenotype was due to the loss of wt- γ-actin function and indicated that drug-resistance phenotype is mediated via altered cross-talk between microtubules and actin.

Altered expression of microtubule-associated protein is also linked to antimicrotubule resistance. Hailat N. et al. (1990) undertaken a quantitative analysis of the major tubulin regulatory protein stathmin by means of two-dimensional gel electrophoresis and revealed that more aggressive neuroblastoma (with high copies of the N-myc gene and less responsive to therapy) have reduced phosphorylation of stathmin.

Further research of cellular structural components by identification of protein isoforms should not only provide valuable insight into the nature of drug resistance mechanisms but also help to develop more successful therapy.

The induction of apoptosis is becoming a popular approach to the treatment of many human cancers, in fact evasion of apoptosis is a key determinant of therapy resistance and neoplastic progression. Over-expression of the protoncogene Bcl-2, found in most neuroblastoma cell lines and in primary neuroblastoma and correlated with a poor prognosis, is reported to be able to block apoptosis induced by some chemotherapeutic agents (cisplatin, doxorubicin and betulinic acid). In the study of Li Y. et al. (2005) the apoptosis and the protein profiles of antisense bcl-2 transfected human neuroblastoma SK-N-MC cells were compared to those of the control cells in order to evaluate the impact of an antisense bcl-2 therapy. Although flow cytometric data revealed that antisense bcl-2 transfection did not cause more extensive apoptosis, the proteomic approach based on 2-DE showed that this treatment induced changes in the expression of various proteins of which seven were identified by N-terminal sequencing. All these proteins were metabolic enzymes except one matched in SWISS-PROT database to the anti-oxidant and anti-apoptosis protein thioredoxin. Based on the authors proposed pathway, up-regulation of thioredoxin may be a result of feedback mechanism induced by Bcl-2 suppression.

Although several mechanisms are responsible for the neuroblastoma multidrug resistance, heterogeneous cell population constituting these solid tumors has been shown to play a great role in the emergence of drug resistance. Sandoval J.A., Eppstein A.C. et al. (2006) investigated proteomic changes associated with resistance or sensitivity to MAPK kinase inhibition in three different neuroblastoma cell phenotypes: SH-SY5Y (N-type), BE (2)-C (I-type) and SK-N-AS (S-type).

Current therapies for neuroblastoma do not use MAPK-directed treatments, but the mitogen activated protein kinase (MAPK) signal transduction pathway is a well-characterized biochemical cascade mediating cell survival and death and is deregulated in a significant proportion of tumors. Several components of this pathway present strategic targets for cancer therapeutic development and the authors investigated whether inhibition of one of the key kinases involved in this pathway (MEK) represents a viable treatment option for neuroblastoma. The three neuroblastoma subtypes were treated with the MEK inhibitor U0126 (10μM) for 1 and 24 hours and analyzed for differential proteins expression by 2-DE. Spots that were down-regulated >2,5-fold after 1h and subsequently up-regulated >5,0-fold after 24h of Mek inhibition were identified by LC-MS/MS. N-type (Mek-resistant) showed the least altered proteomic profile whereas the I-type (MEK-sensitive) and S-type (MEK-intermediate) generated significant protein changes. Identified polypeptides all have roles in mediating an intracellular stress response suggesting that stress related protein expression may be targeted in response to ERK/MAPK therapeutics.

The work of Izbicka E. et al. (2006) reported the presence of differential sensitivity to docetaxel and paclitaxel in the human pediatric tumor xenograft models SK-N-MC and IMR32 (neuroblastoma), RHI and RH30 (rhabdomyosarcoma) and KHOS/NP (osteosarcoma). Six protein species were found by proteomic profiling (four ProteinChip arrays used) to be differentially regulated by docetaxel and paclitaxel in all KHOS/NP xenografts and five proteins in SK-N-MC xenografts. This mass spectrometry analysis could be the first step for the discovery of proteomic biomarkers for drug sensitivity.

Conclusions

The described studies are all useful approaches that will help towards a better understanding of the drug resistance problem by highlighting drug targets and helping in the comprehension of the cellular metabolic pathways involved. Nevertheless we still lack a metanalysis of the overall protein changes, such a data reconstruction will be an absolute requirement to possibly interpret the large amount of the data produced in the proteomics investigations. Moreover the use of cell fractionations and molecules specific tagging would allow to elicit a better view on the drug resistance of Neuroblastoma.

References

Bernardini, S., Bellincampi, L., Ballerini, S., Ranalli, M., Pastore, A., Cortese, C. and Federici, G. (2002). "Role of GST P1-1 in mediating the effect of etoposide on human neuroblastoma cell line Sh-Sy5y." *J. Cell Biochem.* 86(2): 340-7

Brodeur, G.M. (2003). "Neuroblastoma: biological insights into a clinical enigma." *Nat. Rev. Cancer.* 3(3): 203-16

Broker, L.E., Rodriguez J.A., Giaccone G. (2004). *Principles of Molecular Oncology.* 2nd Ed., pp. 463- 489, Humana Press Inc., Totowa, New Jersey

Castel, V., Canete, A., Navarro, S., Garcia-Miguel, P., Melero, C., Acha, T., Navajas, A. and Badal, M.D. (2001). "Outcome of high-risk neuroblastoma using a dose intensity approach: improvement in initial but not in long-term results." *Med. Pediatr. Oncol.* 37(6): 537-42

Chaney, S.G. and Sancar, A. (1996). "DNA repair: enzymatic mechanisms and relevance to drug response." *J. Natl. Cancer Inst.* 88(19): 1346-60

Colabufo, N.A., Berardi, F., Abate, C., Contino, M., Niso, M. and Perrone, R. (2006). "Is the sigma2 receptor a histone binding protein?" *J. Med. Chem.* 49(14): 4153-8

Cole, S.P., Bhardwaj, G., Gerlach, J.H., Mackie, J.E., Grant, C.E., Almquist, K.C., Stewart, A.J., Kurz, E.U., Duncan, A.M. and Deeley, R.G. (1992). "Overexpression of a transporter gene in a multidrug-resistant human lung cancer cell line." *Science.* 258 (5088): 1650-4

Donelli, M.G., Zucchetti, M. and D'Incalci, M. (1992). "Do anticancer agents reach the tumor target in the human brain?" *Cancer Chemother. Pharmacol.* 30(4): 251-60

Erdlenbruch, B., Nier, M., Kern, W., Hiddemann, W., Pekrun, A. and Lakomek, M. (2001). "Pharmacokinetics of cisplatin and relation to nephrotoxicity in paediatric patients." *Eur. J. Clin. Pharmacol.* 57(5): 393-402

Escobar, M.A., Hoelz, D.J., Sandoval, J.A., Hickey, R.J., Grosfeld, J.L. and Malkas, L.H. (2005). "Profiling of nuclear extract proteins from human neuroblastoma cell lines: the search for fingerprints." *J. Pediatr. Surg.* 40(2): 349-58

Figeys, D. (2003). "Proteomics in 2002: a year of technical development and wide-ranging applications." *Anal. Chem.* 75(12): 2891-905

Fisher, D.E. (1994). "Apoptosis in cancer therapy: crossing the threshold." *Cell* 78(4): 539-42

Fountoulakis, M. and Schlaeger, E.J. (2003). "The mitochondrial proteins of the neuroblastoma cell line IMR-32." *Electrophoresis.* 24(1-2): 260-75

Furuta, T., Ueda, T., Aune, G., Sarasin, A., Kraemer, K.H. and Pommier, Y. (2002). "Transcription-coupled nucleotide excision repair as a determinant of cisplatin sensitivity of human cells." *Cancer Res.* 62(17): 4899-902

Gorlick, R., Goker, E., Trippett, T., Steinherz, P., Elisseyeff, Y., Mazumdar, M., Flintoff, W.F. and Bertino, J.R. (1997). "Defective transport is a common mechanism of acquired methotrexate resistance in acute lymphocytic leukemia and is associated with decreased reduced folate carrier expression." *Blood.* 89(3): 1013-8

Gorlick, R., Cole, P., Banerjee, D., Longo, G., Li, W.W., Hochhauser, D. and Bertino, J.R. (1999). "Mechanisms of methotrexate resistance in acute leukemia. Decreased transport and polyglutamylation." *Adv. Exp. Med. Biol.* 457: 543-50

Hailat, N., Strahler, J., Melhem, R., Zhu, X.X., Brodeur, G., Seeger, R.C., Reynolds, C.P. and Hanash, S. (1990). "N-myc gene amplification in neuroblastoma is associated with altered phosphorylation of a proliferation related polypeptide (Op18)." *Oncogene.* 5(11): 1615-8

Hansen, W.K. and Kelley, M.R. (2000). "Review of mammalian DNA repair and translational implications." *J. Pharmacol. Exp. Ther.* 295(1): 1-9

Ishiguro, K., Shyam, K., Penketh, P.G., Sartorelli, A.C. (2005). "Role of O6-alkylguanine-DNA alkyltransferase in the cytotoxic activity of cloretazine." *Mol. Cancer Ther.* 4(11): 1755-63

Ishii, T., Sakurai, T., Usami, H. and Uchida, K. (2005). "Oxidative modification of proteasome: identification of an oxidation-sensitive subunit in 26 S proteasome." *Biochemistry.* 44(42): 13893-901

Izbicka, E., Campos, D., Marty, J., Carrizales, G., Mangold, G. and Tolcher, A. (2006). "Molecular determinants of differential sensitivity to docetaxel and paclitaxel in human pediatric cancer models." *Anticancer Res.* 26(3A): 1983-8

Izquierdo, M.A., Neefjes, J.J., Mathari, A.E., Flens, M.J., Scheffer, G.L. and Scheper, R.J. (1996). "Overexpression of the ABC transporter TAP in multidrug-resistant human cancer cell lines." *Br. J. Cancer.* 74(12): 1961-7

Juliano, R.L. and Ling, V. (1976). "A surface glycoprotein modulating drug permeability in Chinese hamster ovary cell mutants." *Biochim. Biophys. Acta.* 455(1): 152-62

Keshelava, N., Seeger, R.C., Groshen, S. and Reynolds, C.P. (1998). "Drug resistance patterns of human neuroblastoma cell lines derived from patients at different phases of therapy." *Cancer Res.* 58(23): 5396-405

Kubo, T., Kohno, K., Ohga, T., Taniguchi, K., Kawanami, K., Wada, M. and Kuwano, M. (1995). "DNA topoisomerase II alpha gene expression under transcriptional control in etoposide/teniposide-resistant human cancer cells." *Cancer Res.* 55(17): 3860-4

Kushner, B.H., Gilbert, F. and Helson, L. (1986). "Familial neuroblastoma. Case reports, literature review, and etiologic considerations." *Cancer.* 57(9): 1887-93

LaCasse, E.C., Baird, S., Korneluk, R.G. and MacKenzie, A.E. (1998). "The inhibitors of apoptosis (IAPs) and their emerging role in cancer." *Oncogene.* 17(25): 3247-59

Landis, S.H., Murray, T., Bolden, S. and Wingo, P.A. (1999). "Cancer statistics, 1999." *CA Cancer J. Clin.* 49(1): 8-31

Lange, B., Schroeder, U., Huebener, N., Jikai, J., Wenkel, J., Strandsby, A., Wrasidlo, W., Gaedicke, G. and Lode, H.N. (2003). "Rationally designed hydrolytically activated etoposide prodrugs, a novel strategy for the treatment of neuroblastoma." *Cancer Lett.* 197(1-2): 225-30

Li, Y., Lu, Z., Chen, F., Guan, J., Hu, L., Xu, Y. and Chen, J. (2005). "Antisense bcl-2 transfection up-regulates anti-apoptotic and anti-oxidant thioredoxin in neuroblastoma cells." *J. Neurooncol.* 72(1): 17-23

Liebler, D.C., (2002), *Introduction to Proteomics-Tools for the new biology,* pp. 6-8, Humana Press Inc., Totowa, New Jersey

Link, A.J., Eng, J., Schieltz, D.M., Carmack, E., Mize, G.J., Morris, D.R., Garvik, B.M. and Yates, J.R., 3rd (1999). "Direct analysis of protein complexes using mass spectrometry." *Nat. Biotechnol.* 17(7): 676-82

Litman, T., Druley, T.E., Stein, W.D. and Bates, S.E. (2001). "From MDR to MXR: new understanding of multidrug resistance systems, their properties and clinical significance." *Cell Mol. Life Sci.* 58(7): 931-59

Mann, M. and Jensen, O.N. (2003). "Proteomic analysis of post-translational modifications." *Nat. Biotechnol.* 21(3): 255-61

Mora, J., Cheung, N.K., Juan, G., Illei, P., Cheung, I., Akram, M., Chi, S., Ladanyi, M., Cordon-Cardo, C. and Gerald, W.L. (2001). "Neuroblastic and Schwannian stromal cells of neuroblastoma are derived from a tumoral progenitor cell." *Cancer Res.* 61(18): 6892-8

Nakamura, M., Yamada, M., Ohsawa, T., Morisawa, H., Nishine, T., Nishimura, O. and Toda, T. (2006). "Phosphoproteomic profiling of human SH-SY5Y neuroblastoma cells during response to 6-hydroxydopamine-induced oxidative stress." *Biochim. Biophys. Acta.* 1763(9): 977-89

Nasi, S., Ciarapica, R., Jucker, R., Rosati, J. and Soucek, L. (2001). "Making decisions through Myc." *FEBS Lett.* 490(3): 153-62

Oh, J.E., Karlmark, K.R., Shin, J.H., Pollak, A., Freilinger, A., Hengstschlager, M. and Lubec, G. (2005). "Differentiation of neuroblastoma cell line N1E-115 involves several signaling cascades." *Neurochem. Res.* 30(3): 333-48

Pietras, R.J., Fendly, B.M., Chazin, V.R., Pegram, M.D., Howell, S.B. and Slamon, D.J. (1994). "Antibody to HER-2/neu receptor blocks DNA repair after cisplatin in human breast and ovarian cancer cells." *Oncogene.* 9(7): 1829-38

Puchalski, R.B. and Fahl, W.E. (1990). "Expression of recombinant glutathione S-transferase pi, Ya, or Yb1 confers resistance to alkylating agents." *Proc. Natl. Acad. Sci. USA.* 87(7): 2443-7

Reed, J.C., Miyashita, T., Takayama, S., Wang, H.G., Sato, T., Krajewski, S., Aime-Sempe, C., Bodrug, S., Kitada, S. and Hanada, M. (1996). "BCL-2 family proteins: regulators of cell death involved in the pathogenesis of cancer and resistance to therapy." *J. Cell Biochem.* 60(1): 23-32

Rivory, L.P., Slaviero, K.A. and Clarke, S.J. (2002). "Hepatic cytochrome P450 3A drug metabolism is reduced in cancer patients who have an acute-phase response." *Br. J. Cancer.* 87(3): 277-80

Ross, R.A., Biedler, J.L. and Spengler, B.A. (2003). "A role for distinct cell types in determining malignancy in human neuroblastoma cell lines and tumors." *Cancer Lett.* 197(1-2): 35-9

Sandoval, J.A., Eppstein, A.C., Hoelz, D.J., Klein, P.J., Linebarger, J.H., Turner, K.E., Rescorla, F.J., Hickey, R.J., Malkas, L.H. and Schmidt, C.M. (2006). "Proteomic analysis of neuroblastoma subtypes in response to mitogen-activated protein kinase inhibition: profiling multiple targets of cancer kinase signaling." *J. Surg. Res.* 134(1): 61-7

Sandoval, J.A., Hoelz, D.J., Woodruff, H.A., Powell, R.L., Jay, C.L., Grosfeld, J.L., Hickeyd, R.J. and Malkas, L.H. (2006). "Novel peptides secreted from human neuroblastoma: useful clinical tools?" *J. Pediatr. Surg.* 41(1): 245-51

Scheffler, N.K., Miller, S.W., Carroll, A.K., Anderson, C., Davis, R.E., Ghosh, S.S. and Gibson, B.W. (2001). "Two-dimensional electrophoresis and mass spectrometric identification of mitochondrial proteins from an SH-SY5Y neuroblastoma cell line." *Mitochondrion.* 1(2): 161-79

Schiff, P.B., Fant, J. and Horwitz, S.B. (1979). "Promotion of microtubule assembly in vitro by taxol." *Nature.* 277(5698): 665-7

Shimada, H., Ambros, I.M., Dehner, L.P., Hata, J., Joshi, V.V., Roald, B., Stram, D.O., Gerbing, R.B., Lukens, J.N., Matthay, K.K. and Castleberry, R.P. (1999). "The International Neuroblastoma Pathology Classification (the Shimada system)." *Cancer.* 86(2): 364-72

Shin, B.K., Wang, H., Yim, A.M., Le Naour, F., Brichory, F., Jang, J.H., Zhao, R., Puravs, E., Tra, J., Michael, C.W., Misek, D.E. and Hanash, S.M. (2003). "Global profiling of the cell surface proteome of cancer cells uncovers an abundance of proteins with chaperone function." *J. Biol. Chem.* 278(9): 7607-16

Sitek, B., Apostolov, O., Stuhler, K., Pfeiffer, K., Meyer, H.E., Eggert, A. and Schramm, A. (2005). "Identification of dynamic proteome changes upon ligand activation of Trk-receptors using two-dimensional fluorescence difference gel electrophoresis and mass spectrometry." *Mol. Cell Proteomics.* 4(3): 291-9

Smith, M.L. and Seo, Y.R. (2002). "p53 regulation of DNA excision repair pathways." *Mutagenesis.* 17(2): 149-56

Urbani, A., Poland, J., Bernardini, S., Bellincampi, L., Biroccio, A., Schnolzer, M., Sinha, P. and Federici, G. (2005). "A proteomic investigation into etoposide chemo-resistance of neuroblastoma cell lines." *Proteomics.* 5(3): 796-804

Valent, A., Benard, J., Venuat, A.M., Silva, J., Duverger, A., Duarte, N., Hartmann, O., Spengler, B.A. and Bernheim, A. (1999). "Phenotypic and genotypic diversity of human neuroblastoma studied in three IGR cell line models derived from bone marrow metastases." *Cancer Genet. Cytogenet.* 112(2): 124-9

Verrills, N.M., Po'uha, S.T., Liu, M.L., Liaw, T.Y., Larsen, M.R., Ivery, M.T., Marshall, G.M., Gunning, P.W. and Kavallaris, M. (2006). "Alterations in gamma-actin and tubulin-targeted drug resistance in childhood leukemia." *J. Natl. Cancer Inst.* 98(19): 1363-74

Wyllie, A.H. (1997). "Apoptosis and carcinogenesis." *Eur. J. Cell Biol.* 73(3): 189-97

Yu, D., Liu, B., Jing, T., Sun, D., Price, J.E., Singletary, S.E., Ibrahim, N., Hortobagyi, G.N. and Hung, M.C. (1998). "Overexpression of both p185c-erbB2 and p170mdr-1 renders breast cancer cells highly resistant to taxol." *Oncogene.* 16(16): 2087-94

Zeng, H., Chen, Z.S., Belinsky, M.G., Rea, P.A. and Kruh, G.D. (2001). "Transport of methotrexate (MTX) and folates by multidrug resistance protein (MRP) 3 and MRP1: effect of polyglutamylation on MTX transport." *Cancer Res.* 61(19): 7225-32

Zhang, M.H., Lee, J.S., Kim, H.J., Jin, D.I., Kim, J.I., Lee, K.J. and Seo, J.S. (2006). "HSP90 protects apoptotic cleavage of vimentin in geldanamycin-induced apoptosis." *Mol. Cell Biochem.* 281(1-2): 111-21

In: Neuroblastoma Research Trends
Editors: L. H. Andre and N. E. Roux
ISBN: 978-1-60456-790-8

Chapter III

Down Syndrome's Protection Against Neuroblastoma: The Stromal and Neural Overmaturation Tracks

Daniel Satgé[1], Nicole Créau,[2] Revital Aflalo-Rattenbach,[2] Stéphane Ducassou,[3] Patrick Lutz,[3] and Jean Bénard[4]

1. Laboratory of Pathology, Centre Hospitalier, 19012 Tulle, France
2. EA 3508-Université Paris 7, 2 place Jussieu, 75251 Paris, France
3. Pediatric Oncology, CHU Hautepierre, 67098 Strasbourg, France
4. Medical Biology and Pathology Department, UMR-CNRS 8126, Institut Gustave Roussy, 94805 Villejuif, France

Abstract

Strikingly, Down syndrome (DS) or trisomy 21, protects against neuroblastoma. We aimed at understanding the mechanisms involved in this unique constitutional resistance to neural tumors. Indeed, an international epidemiological study conducted in 11 European countries did not find any case of neuroblastoma in children with DS among 6724 young children while more than five were expected [Satgé et al Cancer Research 1998;58:448-52]. Furthermore, only five cases of neuroblastic tumors have been reported so far in children with DS. The protective effect seems specific to peripheral neural tumors and also to central nervous system neural tumors such as medulloblastoma since, conversely, other cancers such as leukaemia, lymphoma, and germ cell tumors are more frequent in children with DS than in the general population. DS phenotype results from the genetic imbalance of the nearly 300 genes mapping to the supernumerary chromosome 21, theoretically up-regulated at a 150% rate through a gene dosage effect. As a matter of fact, adrenal medulla is frequently hypoplastic in children with DS. Several genes located on chromosome 21, expressed in neural and glial tissue may be involved in the reduced incidence of neuroblastoma. They play a role in various functions : apoptosis (ETS2, SOD1, APP), cellular adhesion via direct or indirect effect (DSCAM, CAR, APP), cellular proliferation (ANA, S100B, IFNGR2), anti-angiogenic activity (COL18A1, DSCR1, IFNAR1, IFNAR2, IFNGR2), cellular signalling (ETS2), neural cell maturation and differentiation (S100beta, TIAM1, APP).

We checked three different and complementary cellular approaches. First, *in vitro* growth of neuroblastoma cell lines IGR-N-91, SK-N-SH and SK-N-BE were inhibited by addition of S100B protein in the culture medium, and neuroblasts showed differentiation. Furthermore, the intratumoral injection of S100B in nude mice xenografted with the cell line IGR-N-91 resulted in a 5-10 fold tumor volume reduction compared to control mice. Second, differentiation of the SH-SY-5Y cell line with retinoic acid induced a PCP4 gene expression. Also, in the same cell line, only one additional copy of the PCP4 gene induced a more important and earlier differentiation of these tumoral neuroblasts. Third, the growth of SK-N-AS and SH-SY-5Y cell lines on an extra-cellular matrix (ECM) produced by trisomic 21 fibroblasts was reduced compared to euploid fibroblasts ECM.

These preliminary experiences provide tracks for understanding the striking constitutional resistance to NB in DS and highlight i) an over-maturation state of neural cells and/or ii), the role of extra-cellular molecules produced by Schwann cells and fibroblasts.

Introduction

Neuroblastoma (NB) is the most common extracranial solid tumor in children under 15 years, accounting for nearly 7-10% of childhood cancer, and is the second most solid tumor after central nervous system tumors [Olshan and Bunin 2000, Pearson and Pinkerton 2004]. The prevalence is around 1 case for 7,000 live births. Neuroblastoma, and other neuroblastic tumors such as ganglioneuroblastoma and ganglioneuroma, is derived from the sympathetic nervous system [Pearson and Pinkerton 2004].

The etiology of neuroblastoma is unknown. No causative exogenous agent has been identified. Few studies have suggested the possible role of *in utero* exposure to alcohol, diuretics, seizure medications, fertility drugs or hormones and hair coloring products [Kramer et al 1987, Sasco et al 1998, Olshan and Bunin 2000]. Various parental occupations including farming, painting, electrical works, have been reported in association with neuroblastoma in the offspring. However, there is no consistent evidence of a causative link between the tumor and a particular parental occupation so far. Finally, the potential role of environmental exposures, broadly defined, in the etiology of NB remains quite uncertain [Olsham and Bunin 2000].

Neuroblastoma occurs sporadically. Only one to two percent of patients report a family history of the disease. Then, the tumors occur earlier and are often multiple. Currently, no locus has been identified as the site of a hereditary neuroblastoma gene [Shojaei-Brosseau et al 2004]. Neuroblastoma and other neuroblastic tumors have been found in patients with type 1 neurofibromatosis [Geraci et al 1998], Beckwith-Wiedemann syndrome [Schneid et al., 1997], Hirschsprung disease [Maris et al 1997], and central hypoventilation [Rohrer et atl., 2002].

Additionally, more than 50 various chromosome constitutional anomalies have been reported in children with neuroblastic tumors [Satgé et al 2003a]. A significant part of these anomalies were observed on loci identified as altered in tumoral cells, such as 1p, 2p, 11q and 17q. In NB, the search for a single locus altered similarly to the model of retinoblastoma has failed.

Instead of trying to understand the NB development on the basis of conditions where it is more frequent than in the general population, we have tried here to apply the large current knowledge on NB biology to a condition which protects against neuroblastoma: Down syndrome (DS) (constitutional trisomy 21) [Lejeune et al 1959]. After demonstrating the rarity of NB in DS, we will present some genes of chromosome 21 and their biological effect, which theoretically could explain the reduced incidence of the tumor. Personal preliminary experiences with S100B protein, PCP4 gene, and trisomic 21 fibroblasts extracellular matrix, as well as features of neural and adrenal tissue in DS draw our attention to the neural cell over-differentiation phenomenon, and the role of the extracellular medium. We hypothesize, and provide preliminary experimental evidence, that an earlier and stronger pressure of maturation – differentiation of neural cells, could play a significant role in the protection of persons with DS against NB.

Neuroblastoma Occurs Exceptionally in Children with DS

A review of tumors observed in fetuses, infants, children and adults with constitutional trisomy of chromosomes 8, 9, 13, 18 and 21, revealed a particular distribution of the neoplasms, a kind of "tumor profile" for each syndrome. For a given syndrome, some tumors were observed more frequently than expected [Satgé and Van den Berghe 1996]. A closer attention to the tumor profile of DS through an extensive review of the literature [Satgé et al 1998a] showed, beside an excess of leukaemia and germ cell tumors, a surprisingly small number of neuroblastic tumors with only two neuroblastoma [Miller 1969, Foulkes et al 1997] and one ganglioneuroma [Hosoi et al 1989], while neuroblastoma is the most frequent extracranial solid tumors in young children in the general population [Pearson and Pinkerton 2004]. This lack clearly merges up in previous works on tumors in children with DS [Fabia and Drolette 1970, Narod et al 1991] already reported in a compilation of constitutional anomalies and malformations associated with neuroblastoma [Sy and Edmonson 1968]. Additionally, no child with DS was reported among 1632 neuroblastoma from two series [Miller et al 1968, Neglia et al 1988]. This is surprising since DS, which occurs nearly once every 700 births, is one of the most frequent malformative syndromes. It is well known by pediatricians and usually easily recognized. During the same period hundreds of children with DS have been treated for leukaemia [Narod et al 1991, Dixon et al 2006].

On the basis of these observations, a large epidemiological study was conducted in 11 European countries using childhood cancer registries and neuroblastoma registries (table 1). This study found no child with DS among 6724 children suffering from a neuroblastoma, whereas 5.4 cases were expected on the hypothesis on similar repartition in DS and in the general population. The possible biases such as undeclared DS cases, unrecognized DS cases, under-diagnosed neuroblastoma in children with DS have been considered as unlikely since children were treated by pediatric teams well aware of DS, and since in most of the registries associated conditions are systematically recorded. This result indicates a clear decrease of neuroblastoma incidence in children with DS, and is statistically significant according to the Poisson law ($p=0.0045$) [Satgé et al 1998b].

Table 1. Expected and observed cases of neuroblastoma associated with Down syndrome and Beckwith-Wiedemann syndrome in 6724 neuroblastoma from 11 European countries

Countries	Period covered	Number of neuroblastoma [a]	DS	BW
Denmark	1943-1991	341	0	0
Finland	1985-1994	94	0	0
France	1987-1994	651	0	0
Germany	1979-1995	1398	0	0
Great Britain	1957-1994	2043	0	1
Iceland	1985-1994	3	0	0
Italy	1979-1994	1083	0	0
Netherlands	1970-1995	654	0	2
Norway	1985-1994	86	0	0
Sweden	1985-1994	152	0	0
Switzerland	1971-1995	214	0	1
		6724	0/5.4[b,c]	4/0.5[b]

DS: cases of neuroblastoma associated with Down syndrome.
BW: cases of neuroblastoma associated with Beckwith-Wiedemann syndrome.
a: histologically proved neuroblastoma.
b: first value observed cases, second value expected cases.
c: $p = 0.0045$.

Subsequent studies on neoplasms in children with DS conducted in Japan [Nishi et al 2000], in Denmark [Hasle et al 2000], in Israel [Boker and Merrick 2002], in Finland [Patja et al 2006] and in France [Satgé et al 2003b] did not report a single case of neuroblastoma. Additionally , personal communications, from GM. Brodeur on neuroblastoma registered in the USA, from Z. Mustacchi on a Pediatric Center of Sao Paulo following more than 5000 children with DS, and from WR. Mc Whirter in charge of the Australian Paediatric Cancer Registry indicated no other case in these three large non-European countries. This complementary information indicates that the rarity of neuroblastoma in children with DS is not limited to Europe, but is a worldwide phenomenon. This rarity also applies to the so called neuroblastoma *in situ*. A lesion forty fold more frequent that clinically overt neuroblastoma, and which is usually found at autopsy of fetuses and infant [Mc Williams 1990, Isaacs 1997]. Beside observations of these small tumors in fetuses with Trisomy 13 [Feingold et al 1971, Nevin et al 1972] and in a fetus with trisomy 18 [Robinson et al 1981], only one case has been found in a three-month-infant with DS [Shehata and Abramowsky 2005], although DS is much more frequent than the two other syndromes. In this context it is noteworthy that many fetuses with trisomy 21 have been autopsied during the last decades. It is currently not possible to know the true frequency of neuroblastoma in DS since no case has been reported in a large epidemiological study allowing a calculation. We may only conclude that, although neuroblastoma occurs at a 1/7000 births rate, only 5 cases of neuroblastic tumor [Miller 1969, Hosoi et al 1989, Foulkes et al 1997, Trebo et al 1999, Shehata and Abramowsky 2005] have been recognized and published in individuals with DS who represent a worldly population estimated at 6 millions persons.

Similarly, medulloblastoma, another neural cell embryonnal neoplasm developing in the central nervous system, and which is the most frequent intracranial tumor in childhood [Barger et al 2005] is so rare in DS that it has not been reported until now. However, beside the importantly decreased incidence of neural cell intracranial neoplasms, glial neoplasms do not seem under-represented in children with DS, [Satgé et al 2001b]; it has been even observed in a fetus [Rickert et al 2002]. Thus, it seems that there is in DS a specific decreased incidence of neural cell tumors, both in the central nervous system and in the peripheral nervous system. Neuroblastoma, as well as medulloblastoma, occurs early in life, thus the rarity of these tumors can not be related to a reduced life expectancy. Also, they are probably not related to an exposure to a carcinogenic agent. The protection of persons with DS against these neural neoplasms is more than likely due to a genetic background related to nearly 300 genes mapping to the supernumerary chromosome 21 [Hattori et al 2000, Gardiner et al 2005].

Usually, an impaired genetic background may favor cancer development. This is observed in children with type 1 neurofibromatosis, with beckwith-Wiedemann syndrome, with tuberous sclerosis, with Gorlin syndrome and with Turcot syndrome for instance [Stiller 2005]. However, we have precisely here a situation where a constitutional genetic imbalance (i.e. Down syndrome) protects against a given neoplasm (i.e. neuroblastoma), whereas other types of cancers such as leukaemia and testicular tumors are unquestionably increased.

This very unusual situation (according to the current knowledge) is a rare opportunity of a natural model of protection against a cancer. As such, it bears the cellular and tissular mechanisms that we should try to understand, and if possible that we should use to fight against neuroblastoma. This prompted us to look for in what the neural cell of peripheral nervous system in DS is so remarkably reluctant to neoplastic transformation.

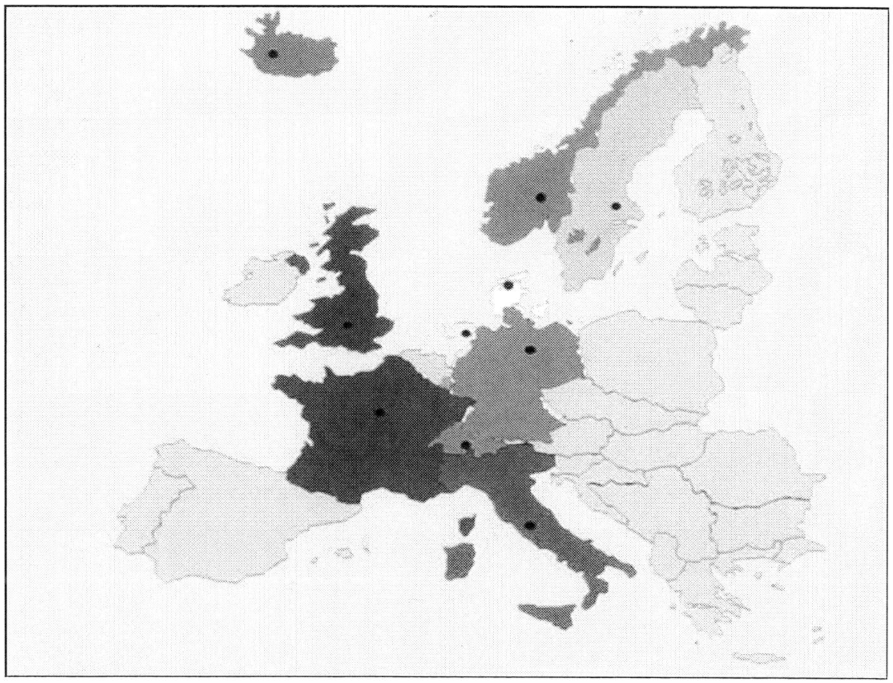

Figure 1. No case of Down syndrome was found among 6724 neuroblastoma in eleven European countries.

Analysis of the Cases of Neuroblastic Tumors Reported in Infants and Children with DS

A closer look at the few observations of neuroblastic tumors in children with DS reveals interesting features.

A first case of neuroblastoma, in a 5-month-old male infant, was reported in an epidemiological study on congenital malformations associated with cancer during the years 1960-1966 in the USA [Miller 1969]. The localization of the tumor is not given. At that time, the group of small round cell tumors of childhood was not well known and immunohistochemistry labelling was not available [Joshi et al 2000]. Thus, a little doubt about the true nature of this tumor remains. For instance, an Ewing tumor, which may present with very close histological features with neuroblastoma, cannot be excluded. However, if so, this case would have to be retained as the first example. On the contrary, a more recent report of a lumbar paravertebral grade 4 neuroblastoma in a 12-year-old Japanese boy is really doubtful [Koyama et al 1999]. We do not consider it is a neuroblastoma given the following points. The patient was more than 10 years old while neuroblastoma occurs mainly before 5 years of age; there was no biologic serum or tissular marker of neuroblastoma and particularly no 1p deletion, despite the bad histological aspect of the tumor. Additionally, the tumor did not respond to a treatment directed against neuroblastoma [Satgé et al 2001a, Satgé et al 2003a]. In our point of view it could be another kind of small blue cell tumor of childhood, and particularly an Ewing tumor which may be observed in the paravertebral region [Hariyama et al 2003]. Indeed, Ewing tumor occurs in children with DS [Miller 1969, Satgé et al 2003b]. In fact, recent data indicate that Ewing tumor is not developed from a neural precursor, but originates from a mesenchymal stem cell [Tirode et al 2006]. Such an evidence fits well with the fact that neural tumors are very rare in DS, while mesenchymal tumors seem to be over-represented, particularly in the central nervous system [Satgé et al 2001b].

A second case was reported in a study on associated congenital anomalies in a series of French-Canadian children with neuroblastoma [Foulkes et al 1997]. It was an undebatable stage 3 neuroblastoma of the left adrenal in a 15-month-old female infant who had a good outcome after treatment (Dr J. Foulkes personal communication). The third case is a stage 4 neuroblastoma of the left adrenal in a 19-month-old Canadian black boy which has been reported twice, since the child later developed an acute plasmatic interstitial nephritis [Al-Herni et al 1999, Trebo et al 1999]. This case is particularly noteworthy since the child responded unusually well to the treatment of chemotherapy and radiotherapy despite of the presence of several adverse prognostic factors. It is a rare example of treatment success in a stage 4 neuroblastoma. The authors speculated that an over-expression of the S100B gene contributed to the long term survival of the child [Trebo et al 1999].

Besides these three cases of neuroblastoma, two other neuroblastic tumors have been published. A ganglioneuroma of the left sympathetic ganglia was removed from the retroperitoneal region in a 6-year-old Japanese boy with mosaic DS (46XY/47XY, +21) [Hosoi et al 1989]. The outcome is not known. As the child was not homogeneous for trisomy 21, we wonder if the population of euploid cells could not have favored the neoplasm, by lowering the possible anti-neoplastic effect of trisomy 21 against neuroblastic tumors. The fifth and last case is an *in situ* neuroblastoma discovered at the autopsy of a 3-month-old male infant with DS who died from alveolar capillary dysplasia [Shehata and Abramowsky 2005]. It must be kept in mind that *in situ* neuroblastoma are precursors of neuroblastoma, and are nearly forty times more frequent than overt neuroblastoma. They usually spontaneously regress and are frequently associated with congenital anomalies [Shanklin and Sotelo-Avila 1969, Isaacs 1997]. In this last case, we wonder whether the genetic background which leads to the associated disease could not have also favored the onset of the small neoplasm against the protective background of DS.

Thus, our analysis of these five cases of neuroblastic tumors is that two neoplasms could have been related to a particular situation (constitutional chromosome mosaicism and congenital associated malformative disease), while two others are true stage 3 and stage 4 neuroblastoma who responded unusually well to treatment. In conclusion, beside hundreds cases of leukemias found in children with DS [Yang et al 2002, Dixon et al 2006] only five neuroblastic tumors have been reported, two having an unusually good outcome. This review strengthens the concept that constitutional trisomy 21 protects against neuroblastoma, not only by reducing the occurrence of the tumor, but also by allowing a better outcome after usual treatments.

Aspects of Adrenal Medulla in DS

Adrenal medulla is the most frequent site of origin for neuroblastoma. Histological features of this gland in DS, where neuroblastic tumors are unusually rare, could provide indications for understanding the mechanism involved in the protection. Adrenal medulla is derived from cells of the neural crest of the embryon [Mora and Gerald 2004] which mix with the future cortical cells at six weeks, and gather in the center of the gland at 15 weeks [Turkel and Itabashi 1974]. At seven weeks, appear sustentacular cells which are well seen using antibodies directed against S100B protein [Cooper et al 1990, Magro and Grasso 1997]. These cells will be found in the center of the islets of neuroblasts. The fetal medulla remains small until birth, a time when it accounts for only 1% of the weight of the gland and consist of a thin plate of immature neuroblasts. After the second month post-natally, maturation takes place, and at four months the adrenal medulla is composed mainly of mature cells and sustentacular cells, neuroblasts being scarce. Then, the medulla will grow, faster until 3 years of age, and slower later to account for nearly 10% of the weight of the gland in early adulthood [Kreiner 1982]. During all this development process and later, neuroblasts and mature adrenal cells are in close contact with the sustentacular cells without separation by a basal lamina (Iwanaga and Fujita 1984). Unfortunately, as far as we are aware, data on adrenal medullary development in DS is not available yet. Only a recent immunohistochemical evaluation of S100B protein of infants with DS aged one day to two years studied adrenals and found no differences in the distribution of sustentacular cells compared to non-trisomic infants [Michetti et al 1990].

Adrenals have been poorly studied in DS. However, in the early 20th century, and particularly in the thirties, the idea of a possible endocrine genesis of DS has been the subject of much investigation and discussion leading to a more detailed examination of endocrine glands [Gordon 1930]. Our search in the literature found, beside rare reports where adrenal medullary was considered as normal [Pennacchietti 1935, Tatafiore 1937 case 2], five publications describing an atrophic or absent adrenal medullary tissue (table 2). The reduction in size was observed after the first months of life [Lhermitte et al 1921, Gordon 1930]. Since adrenal medulla is difficult to see, particularly in young infants, and necessitates well orientated histological slides from the center of the gland it is possible that some histologists, having some doubt about their histological preparations could hesitate before reporting an hypoplasia. We will have to wait for Benda in 1960 [Benda 1960] to have a clear description of theses anomalies. Worthnoting is the fact that, in a first publication on endocrine aspects of mongolism in 1942 based on 38 autopsies, Benda wrote "the medulla appears to be well developed" [Benda 1942].

These discrepancies from literature clearly show us the difficulties of histological examination of this gland. Nonetheless, according to his most recent study based on 44 autopsies of subjects with DS from birth to adulthood, medullary cells "were sparse in many cases". The author adds "few showed hypertrophy with considerable amount of fibrosis". According to Benda, medullary function is inadequate on account of the insufficient development of the chromaffin cells [Benda 1960]. Benda described also a population of eosinophil cells and a large zone between cortex and medullary (the usual X zone well observed in animals) which is not usually seen in human. As far as we are aware after Benda's works no histological general study on adrenal medulla in DS is available.

Obviously a study with current means such as electronic microscopy and immunohistochemistry on the morphological aspects of adrenal medulla is needed to provide more precise data on the following points: frequency, importance and descriptive features of the adrenal medulla hypoplasia in subjects with DS. Interestingly, these first observations are in agreement with physiopathological studies that found a defect in sympathetic nervous response to various forms of stress in individuals with DS [Eberhard et al 1991]. The lower values of adrenalin in urine, despite normal serum values, indicate a reduction of liberation of adrenalin from adrenal medulla [Lake et al 1979]. These data has been seriously considered to explain the reduced response to stress in persons with DS. However, things are not so simple since, on the other hand, adrenergic response seems to be either enhanced or reduced in various trisomic cells [McSwigan et al 1981, Sheppard et al 1983, Fernhall and Otterstetter 2003].

Table 2. Cases of adrenal medulla hypoplasia and aplasia in subjects with Down syndrome reported in the literature

Authors	Age and sex	Medical history	Aspect of adrenal medulla at autopsy
Lange 1906	F, 8 years	Croup, bronchopneumonia	Nearly no adrenal tissue
Lhermitte et al 1921	M, 3 months	Diarrhoea	Adrenal medulla replaced by connective tissue and dilated vessels. Absence of chromaffin cells
Gordon 1930 Case 1	F, 14 months	Bronchopneumonia	Poorly developed medulla, hypoplasia of chromaffin cells
Gordon 1930 Case 2	F, 6 weeks	Malnutrition, pylorospasm	Rare *islets* of medullary cells
Delfini 1932	M, 8 years	Miliary tuberculosis	Complete medullary aplasia, no chromaffin cells
Tatafiore 1937 Case 1	M, 3 months	Bronchopneumonia	Slight hypoplasia of adrenal medulla
Benda 1960	44 patients, F and M, children and adults	Not available	Adrenal medullas of irregular size, rare medullary cells. Rare hypertrophic medullas with abundant fibrosis

Beside the reduced number of cells in the adrenal medullary, histological studies of the peripheral nervous tissue of various organs in DS have also showed a reduced number of neural cells. The number of neurons in the ganglia of the deep submucous and Auerbach plexuses of the oesophagus is reduced to nearly three-fourths of normal values [Nakazato et al 1986]. Also, the quantitative morphometric study of the ventral cochlear nucleous of the peripheral auditory system showed, in infant with DS, a greatly reduced number of neurons [Gandolfi et al 1981]. Furthermore, it has been suggested that tooth agenesis in persons with DS could be related to fewer nerves and fewer nerve branches [Russel and Kjaer 1995].

These works indicate that the quantitative reduction of neural cells is not limited to the adrenal medullary, but is observed in various parts of the peripheral nervous system. Furthermore, there is in the brain of Down syndrome subjects a reduced gray matter volume [Pearlson et al 1998] and decreased neuronal density in some areas [Sylvester 1983, Casanova et al 1985, Pine et al 1997, Buxhoeveden et al 2002]. Thus, it seems to result from a general mechanism particular to DS. The mechanism leading to reduced neural cells in the peripheral and central nervous system is unknown so far. It could result from an abnormal cell death, for instance by increased apoptosis or a default in production of these cells by negative cell control and premature neural cell maturation. According to Pine and colleagues [Pine et al 1997] who studied the inferior olivary neuron number in DS, the reduced number of neural cells, similarly to other brain areas results from reduced initial neural production rather than post natal loss. We hypothetize that this reduced production is related to enhanced and abnormally precocious neural cell differentiation which will impair normal cell division.

Genes on Chromosome 21 which could Protect Against Neural Cancer and Particularly Neuroblastoma

DS phenotype is due to a constitutional trisomy of chromosome 21 [Lejeune et al 1959]. Human chromosome 21, the smallest of our autosomes, contains around 300 genes [Hattori et al 2000, Gardiner et al 2005], nearly 1% of the human genome. DS phenotype includes a facial dysmorphism, an intellectual disability of variable severity, congenital malformations, mainly of the heart and digestive tract, and various organ and tissue impairments. It has been evaluated that more than 80 clinical features occur more frequently than in the general population [Cohen 1999]. These features, which are seen with variable severity, are not unique to persons with constitutional trisomy 21, but also occur in the general population [Epstein 2001].

The phenotype of DS is a consequence of the genetic imbalance related to the genes on the supernumerary chromosome 21 [Epstein 1990, Korenberg et al 1994]. According to the gene dosage effect hypothesis, triplicated genes are overexpressed at a rate of 150% in all cells, and the phenotype is a direct result of triplicated loci [Epstein 1988]. Although until now it has not been proved that a particular phenotype feature is related to a single gene dosage effect, it is considered that this mechanism could explain some aspects of DS. In fact, it is now clear that genes on chromosome 21 and their products interfere between them and also with genes situated on other chromosomes in various cells and tissues [Fitzpatrick 2005, Roper and Reeves 2006]. Furthermore, the process is time (*i.e.* during development or after maturation) and space (*i.e.* in different tissues) dependent. Thus, DS is a very complex genetic condition. One promising concept roots in the observation that some genes on chromosome 21 interact with particular biochemical pathways [Gardiner 2003] leading to a given phenotype consequence. For a better understanding of these preferential pathways a good knowledge of the effect of genes on chromosome 21 is needed. We here report here some data dealing with genes of chromosome 21 which act on neural tissue and could have a protecting role against neural neoplasms.

Apoptosis and other degenerative processes leading to cell death have an antineoplastic role by reducing the number of tumoral cells, thus lowering the burden of tumoral tissue. Selective neural, but not glial, apoptosis related to oxidative stress, and increased intracellular reactive oxygen species have been reported in DS [Busciglio and Yankner 1995]. The ETS2 gene (homologue of the ets sequence of the avian retrovirus E26), mapping to chromosome 21 and overexpressed in neural cells of persons with DS, leads to increased apoptosis [Wolvetang et al 2003]. This effect is probably related to an increased flux of oxygen peroxide due to an over-expression of another gene mapping to chromosome 21: SOD1 (for Cu/Zn Superoxide Dismutase 1) [Ceballos-Picot et al 1991, de Haan et al 1996]. Other genes on chromosome 21 such as S100B (for S-100 calcium – binding protein, beta chain) [Hu et al 1997], APP (for Amyloid Protein Precursor) [Shaked et al 2006] and DSCR1 (for Down Syndrome Candidate Region 1), a regulator of calcineurin [Fuentes et al 2000] which are expressed in neural tissue have also been thought to be implicated in neurodegeneration.

Alterations in the process of cell adhesion may lead to neoplastic transformation. Furthermore, experimental restauration of normal adhesion between cells and with their micro-environment has been sufficient to reverse the neoplastic transformation in some tumors [Spiryda et al 1998]. Among the genes acting on cell adhesion mapping to chromosome 21: DSCAM, CAR and APP are of interest. The Down Syndrome Cell Adhesion Molecule (DSCAM), a member of the superfamily of cell adhesion molecules, is expressed in developing neurons of the central and peripheral nervous system, including neural crest derivatives [Barlow et al 2002]. The gene for Coxsackievirus and Adenovirus Receptor (CAR) is expressed in neural cells, mainly during development. It has been found at least in the NB cell line SH-SY5Y [Skog et al 2002]. APP also favors cell-cell and cell-substrate adhesion, as observed with the Neuro-2A NB cell line [Breen et al 1991]. An over-production of the corresponding proteins could induce neuroblast migration anomalies during embryogenesis and fetal life. Later, such an over-production could lead neural cells to a more resistant state to oncologic transformation.

Angiogenesis plays an important role in NB development, and a spectrum of stimulators and inhibitors of angiogenesis have been detected in NB tumors [Ribatti et al 2006]. At least, five genes mapping to chromosome 21 have an anti-angiogenic power: DSCR1, COL18A1, IFNAR1, IFNAR2, IFNGR2. *In vivo*, the over expression of DSCR1 reduces angiogenesis through a negative feedback loop with the vascular endothelial growth factor (VEGF) [Abe and Sato 2001, Minami et al 2004]. It is noteworthy that VEGF correlates with MYCN expression and with the growth of NB [Marcus et al 2005]. Endostatin, the clivage product of collagen XVIII gene (COL18A1) is a powerful inhibitor of tumor-induced angiogenesis also expressed in NB [Kuroiwa et al 2003]. Serum levels of endostatin are significantly more elevated in persons with DS than in persons without DS. It has been suggested that this over-production could inhibit solid tumors development [Zorick et al 2001]. Three genes coding for receptors of the interferon system: Interferon Alpha Receptor 1 (IFNAR1), Interferon Alpha Receptor 2 (IFNAR2) and Interferon Gamma Receptor 2 (IFNGR2) are localized on chromosome 21 [Gardiner 2003]. Furthermore, trisomic 21 cells are much more sensitive than euploid cells to human interferon [Tan et al 1974]. Since IFN-alpha, IFN-beta and IFN-gamma have the power to reduce, by inhibition of tumor-induced angiogenesis, the proliferation of various xenografted NB cells lines [Streck et al 2004, Ribatti et al 2006], it is very likely that the corresponding receptor genes also have a protective effect against NB proliferation in infants with DS.

An antiproliferative action of genes on chromosome 21 expressed in neural cells has been identified, at least for BTG3, IFN gamma and S100B. BTG3 gene (for B-cell Translocation Gene-3) also named ANA (for Abundant in Neuroepithelium Area) is a member of a newly identified family of antiproliferative genes expressed in the developing nervous system. It could have an overlapping role with BTG2 in the growth arrest of neural precursor cells at a time when the commitment of the precursor cells to the neural or glial lineage occurs [Yoshida et al 1998, El-Ghissassi et al 2002]. ANA impairs the cycle cell progression in NIH3T3 cells [Yoshida et al 1998]. Importantly, IFN gamma already cited above, has beside its immuno-regulatory and anti-angiogenic activities, a strong anti-proliferative effect on NB tumor cells [Airoldi et al 2004]. Previously, it was observed an inhibition of growth of the NB cell line B104 using S100B protein, (the product of S100B gene) at concentrations which stimulate glial cell proliferation [Selinfreund et al 1991]. Since cycle cell arrest is known to be an essential preliminary requirement for terminal differentiation, we may also consider that these four genes, and possibly others inhibiting the cycle cell, prepare the first step of neural cell differentiation.

Differentiation – maturation is a process which lowers tumoral aggressiveness, and, at most may lead to tumor involution. This is particularly true for embryonal tumors such as neuroblastoma which express the potency of the embryonic primordium [Kissane 1994]. It is thus important to bear in mind that, to cite only three genes on chromosome 21, S100B, TIAM1 and APP are involved in neural differentiation. It has been shown that S100B protein, produced by glial cells in the central nervous system and by Schwann cells in the peripheral nervous system, besides its cytotoxic action and its role in growth inhibition, stimulates the outgrowth of neural cells [Winningham-Major et al 1989]. Interestingly, the murine NB cell line Neuro-2a reacts by extending neurites in the presence of S100B protein in the extra-cellular medium [Kligman and Hsieh 1987]. TIAM1 (for T-Lymphoma Invasion and Metastasis gene 1), a specific guanine nucleotide exchange factor for Rac1, is involved in the neurite outgrowth, particularly observed in the NB cell line NB1. It locates downstream the Ephrin-B1 or EphA2 mediated signalling [Tanaka et al 2004]. APP has been shown to stimulate neurite outgrowth [Qiu et al 1995, Allinquant et al 1995]. Also its phosphorylation has been shown to play a role during neuronal differentiation in PC12 [Ando et al 1999]. But, due to the numerous protein products generated through transcription and post-translational modification, different physiological roles of APP are expected [for review Zheng and Koo 2006].

In this brief review it was not possible to cite all the genes known on chromosome 21, more or less directly implicated in neural cell biology related to carcinogenesis. This would necessitate more space, and is beyond the scope of this chapter. For instance, it is known that in DS, the immune system is deficient while at least eight genes working for the immune response have been identified on chromosome 21 [Gardiner 2003]. This leads to a higher susceptibility to infections. However, the repercussions of the immune dysregulation on malignancies of persons with DS are not known. Although we have artificially separated the different types of action of the various genes, these actions are related. For instance, growth inhibition is a first step for tissue differentiation, and cell adhesion itself may promote neurite growth. Furthermore, a single gene and its product is sometimes implicated in different cellular responses. For instance, S100B protein is both cytotoxic at high concentration for PC12 cell line, growth inhibiting for primitive neural cells and NB cell lines, and a differentiating protein for NB cells on other experimental conditions. IFN gamma has both an antiproliferative action on NB cell lines and an inhibitory effect on tumor-induced angiogenesis. ETS2, besides its role on apoptosis can also, when over-expressed, reverse the tumoral phenotype induced by RAS oncogene [Foos et al 1998]. APP through its different protein products has been shown to interfere at least with cell adhesion, cell differentiation and neurodegeneration. Considering all these data and the complex known and unknown interactions of genes of chromosome 21 and their products, it is particularly difficult to predict how a neural trisomic cell will react to the genetic imbalance in the field of oncogenesis. An interesting approach would be to consider precisely the final phenotype of a tissue, particularly at morphological and biochemical levels since it is accepted that an experimental system alone, whether cell cultures or mouse models, will be sufficient to unravel genes-pathway-phenotype correlates in DS [Gardiner 2003, Ma'ayan et al 2006].

Personal data: 1. S100 B inHibits the Growth of Neuroblastoma Cell Lines *in Vitro* and *in Vivo*

S100B protein, extracted from bovine brain forty years ago [Moore 1965] is the product of S100B gene mapping to 21q22.3 [Allore et al 1990]. S100B is a main member of the S100 family which accounts for the largest group of the E-F hand protein superfamily [Marenholz et al 2004]. This 10.5 kDa dimeric (two beta chains) soluble acidic protein contains two different E-F hands. Upon Ca^{2+} binding S100B undergoes a conformational change with exposure of a hydrophobic surface where bound various target proteins. S100B is the major S100 protein in the brain, constitutionally secreted at low levels by astrocytes. It is also produced by Schwann cells, and in sustentacular cells in the adrenal medulla [Michetti et al 1990, Magro and Grasso 1997]. S100B acts intracellularly on Ca^{2+} homeostasis, cytoskeletal organisation and transcription in a Ca^{2+} dependant manner [Donato 1999, Donato 2003]. In the extracellular space S100B binds to the receptor for advanced glycation end products (RAGE). Its paracrine effects exhibit a neurotrophic activity, while autocrine effects are a stimulation of glial proliferation [Selinfreund et al 1991, Huttunen et al 2000]. In transgenic mice increased expression of S100B in the brain stimulates astrogliosis and neurite proliferation. The mice show enhanced exploratory activity, reduced anxiety, but also impaired learning and memory as well as altered synaptic plasticity [Marenholz et al 2004]. Conversely, knock out mice exhibit more neural plasticity and enhanced spatial memory [Nishiyama et al 2002].

Interestingly, studies on S100B in NB have shown that abundant amount of protein in tumoral tissue is correlated with a much better survival of patients, even in poorly differentiated NB, and even in patients over two years of age [Misugi et al 1985, Shimada et al 1985, Hachitanda et al 1992, Nagoshi et al 1992]. Four previous experiments have evaluated the effect of S100B protein on NB cell lines, but not in the context of an antineoplastic action. The first revealed neurite extension after 2 to 6 hours with purified S100B at doses 300 ng/ml on the neuro-2A cell line [Kligman and Hsieh 1987]. The second, using VUSB1 recombinant S100B at doses 30 ng/ml, found a 48% reduced cellularity after two days of culture on the same NB cell line [Selinfreund et al 1991]. A third one using purified S100AB protein at doses 10µg/ml describes a 20% reduced cellularity and apoptosis in the GICAN NB cell line after five days of culture [Fano et al 1993]. Finally, a coculture of astrocytes and the B104 NB cell line with VUSB1 recombinant S100B at doses 60µg/ml leaded to 34% cell death and 16% apoptosis after two days of culture [Hu et al 1997]. However the experiments were for most of them briefly reported and conducted in murine cell line except for GIKAN. This prompted us to evaluate the effect of S100B protein on three human cell lines.

Aiming at evaluating the effect of S100B protein on human NB we have used three NB cell lines: SK-N-SH [Biedler et al 1973] which is a poorly aggressive NB cell line, SK-N-BE [Biedler et al 1976] and IGR-N-91 [Ferrandis et al 1994] which are two highly aggressive NB cell lines with 1p deletion and N-MYC amplification [Thiele 1999]. As indicated in a previous report [Satgé 1996] cells were grown on slides 22x22 mm in 6-well plates at a density varying between 1000 and 14000 cells / cm^2. At initial plating and every two days 25 ng to 1000 ng S100B/ml were added to the medium (bovine brain S100B protein Sigma # S.8390). Cells were counted with a light microscopic equipped with a square grid after staining with Mayer's Hemalun and mounting the slides. For all cell lines, a growth inhibition varying from 20% to more than 70%, compared to controls was observed for a concentration of S100B of 50 ng or more per 1000 cells plated. This inhibition was not observed when fibroblasts were grown in the same condition [see Satgé 1996]. The inhibiting effect was often observed early during the first day of culture. Histologically we observed both cells showing involution and cells showing neurite extension which indicated a process of differentiation.

After the encouraging results of *in vitro* experiences using NB cell lines it was decided to evaluate the effect of S100B protein in a xenograft model of an aggressive NB cell line: IGR-N-91. This cell line originates from medullary metastases of a stage 4 neuroblastoma developed in an 8-year-old by who died from a relapse of his neoplasm. It is a typical immature NB characterized by N-MYC amplification and 1p deletion [Ferrandis et al 1994]. Similarly to *in vitro* experiences we used S100B protein extracted and purified from bovine brain. Bovine S100B is very close to human S100B [Zimmer et al 1995]. Animals were female athymic Swiss mice bred in the animal experimentation unit at the Institut Gustave Roussy (Villejuif, France). Experiences were carried out on accordance with the animal protection and hygiene condition established by the European Community (Directive 86/609/CEE). 18 mice 6-8 weeks of age were injected in the left side a 0.2 ml suspension of 2.5 x 10^6 tumoral cells, and were randomly assigned in three groups. When most of the animals presented a visible nodule at the site of the xenograft (*i.e.* 34 days following the graft), mice were given S100B by intratumoral injections; finaly, 14 injections of 0.2 ml were given at this place, every two days during a total period of four weeks. The first group (control) received the vehicle alone , the second group received 300 ng of S100B protein at each injection, and the third group received 30μg of S100B protein at each injection. At the end of the program, animals were autopsied, fresh xenograft tissue specimen were fixed with formalin, cut in 3 mm pieces, embedded in paraffin and routinely stained with hematoxylin an eosin. The tumor volumes were estimated and the mean values of each group were compared see figure 2.

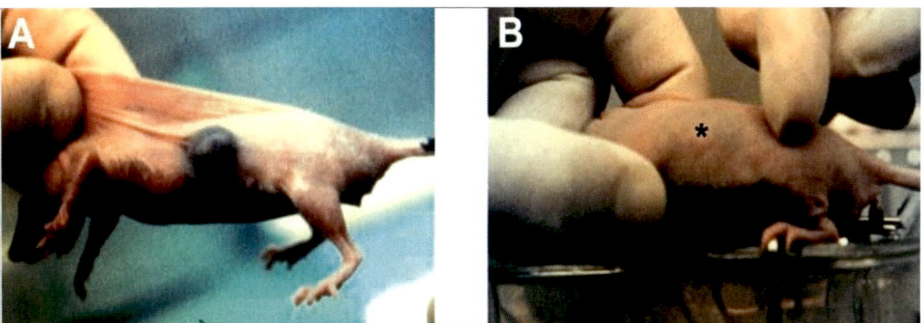

Figure 2. Aspect of the flank of nude mice which received a xenograft of IGR-N-91 neuroblastoma cell line. Animals received either PBS (Dulbecco L w/o Ca^{++}-Mg^{++}, Seromed) 0.9 mM calcium and phosphate buffer KH_2 PO_4 to obtain a pH at 6.4 according to Selinfreund et al 1991 (for the control group). The same preparation containing 300 ng or 30 µg of S100B protein was injected respectively in groups 2 and 3. 2A: Animal in the control group, 2B: animal which received 14 injections of 300 ng of S100B protein.

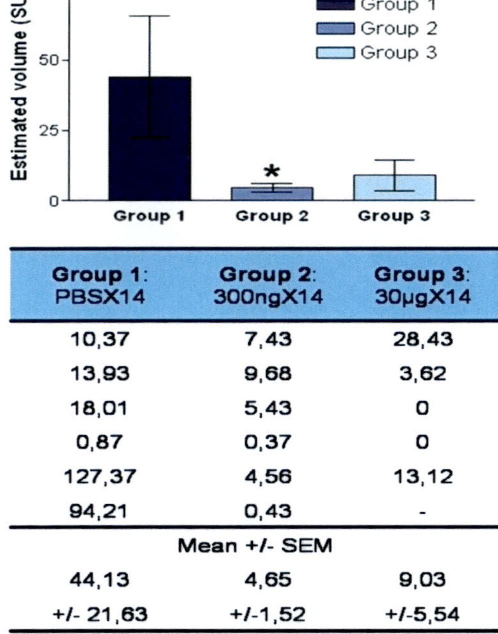

Group 1: PBSX14	Group 2: 300ngX14	Group 3: 30µgX14
10,37	7,43	28,43
13,93	9,68	3,62
18,01	5,43	0
0,87	0,37	0
127,37	4,56	13,12
94,21	0,43	-
	Mean +/- SEM	
44,13	4,65	9,03
+/- 21,63	+/-1,52	+/-5,54

Figure 3. Effect of S100B on IGR-N-91 neuroblastoma cell line xenograft. For the smallest tumors, the volume was estimated by adding the measured tumoral surfaces observed with a light microscope equipped with a square gird of all the slides separated from 3 mm.

In the control group, the mean estimated volume was 44.13 SU (surface unit) (SEM =21.63). For group 2, of animals which received 300 ng of S100B protein the mean estimated volume was 4.65 SU (SEM = 1.52). In group 3 receiving 30 µg S100B the estimated volume was 9.03 SU, (SEM = 5.54) (fig 3). Due to the high variability of the volume distribution, the Bartlett's statistical test was used. This test shows a statistically significant difference between the estimated volume of tumors of the control group (group 1) and group 2. In group 2 the mean volume is 10 fold smaller than in the control group (p = 0.05). In group 3, tumors are 5 fold smaller than is the control group, but the result is not statistically significant given the large variability. However it is important to notice that the only two mice which did not had a tumor at the end of the experience were from group 3 of animals receiving the highest dose of S100B protein (figure 3).

For the largest tumors, it was estimated that, given their visible shape, the tumors were a sphere with a central area being $S= \pi r^2$ and adjacent areas are $S_1= S-\pi d^2$ ("r" being the radius and "d" being the distance between each section, *i.e.*,3 mm), and their volume values were obtained in summing the tumor surfaces. The results of estimated volume were given in surface unit (SU) (*) variances differ significantly ($p<0.05$) according to Bartlett's test for equal variances.

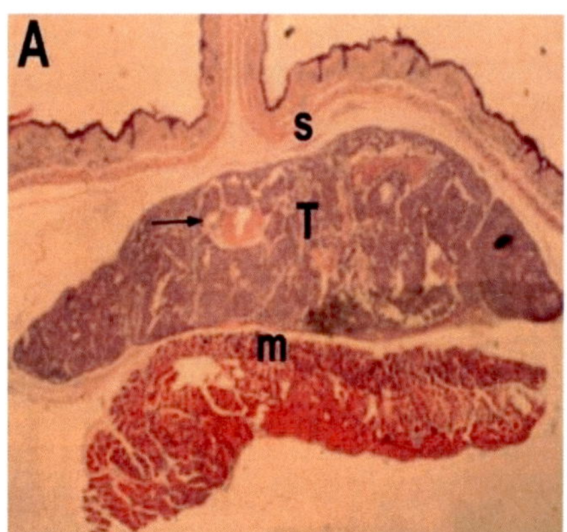

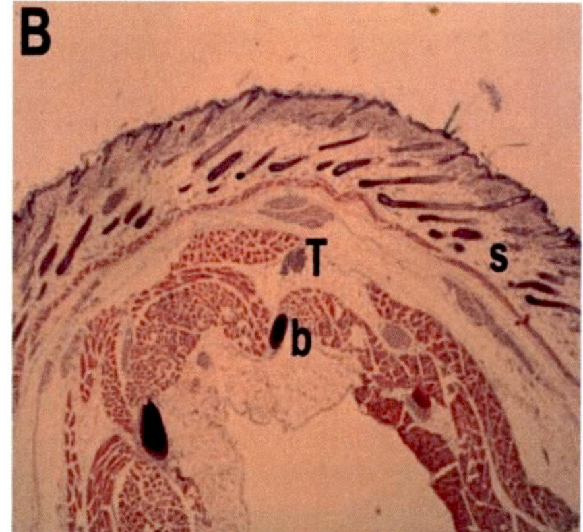

Figure 4. Histological preparations (HE,x20) of the flank of a mouse in the control group (4A) with a large subcutaneous tumor and a very small tumor in a mouse of the group which received the low doses: 300 ng S100B protein (4B) One animal in group 3 was excluded from the study: it is the only one which had already a large tumor at the beginning of S100B protein injections.

At the histological level (figure 4) no difference was observed between small and large tumors. Interestingly, we did not observe an excess of necrosis or apoptosis, particularly in tumors of group 2 and of group 3.

Another study was conducted using animals xenografted with the same IGR-N-91 cell line in the right side and cutaneous injection in the left side. This experience showed no difference in the volume distribution between mice receiving S100B or PBS only.

Data obtained from these experiments indicate that S100B protein inhibits NB cell line growth *in vitro*. It also inhibits a xenograft of a highly aggressive NB cell line *in vivo* according to our preliminary trial.

Personal Data: 2. PCP4 Induces Earlier Neuroblastoma Differentiation

The PCP4 (Purkinje Cell Protein-4) genes are localized on human chromosome 21 and on mouse chromosome 16 [Cabin et al 1996] and encode a protein also named PEP-19 [Chen and Orr 1990]. This protein is a Ca++-calmodulin modulator, also called calpacitin [Gerendasy 1999] or camstatin [Slemmon et al 1996]. *Pcp4* has been shown to be expressed in a subset of neurons, namely Purkinje cerebellar neurons with increasing expression from post-natal stage up to adult stage [Sangameswaran et al 1989]. First described to be strictly neuronal, mouse embryogenesis studies have shown a wider expression namely in ectoderm, neuroectoderm and neural crest derived cells. The transcripts are mainly observed in post-mitotic cells [Thomas et al 2003]. The PCP4 protein (PEP-19) is a 61aa IQ motif protein containing several serine residues that may be phosphorylated by cAMP-dependent kinase (PKA) and Mitogen-Activated Kinases [Slemmon et al 1996]. Phosphorylation is suggested to regulate binding to apo-CaM as for the two other camstatins : neurogranin (RC-3) and neuromodulin (GAP-43). Recently, it has been shown that the serine close to the IQ sequence is phosphorylated by PKCs and that this phosphorylation induces a lower affinity to CaM [Dickerson et al 2006].

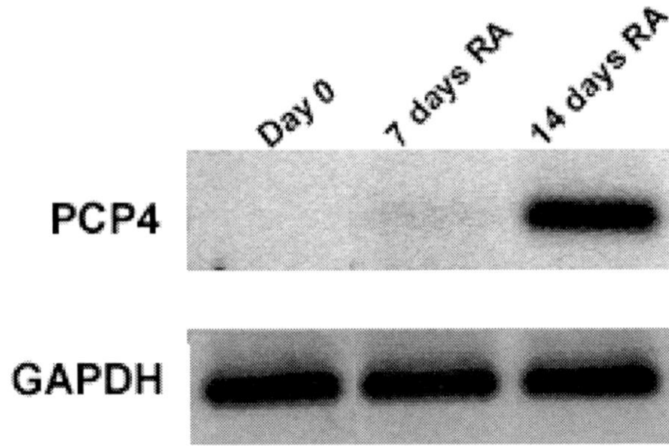

Figure 5. Expression of the human PCP4 gene in the SH-SY5Y cells during RA-induced differentiation. GAPD (Glyceraldehyde 3 phosphate dehydrogenase) is used as reference.

Insights into the function of PCP4 have been brought through several studies. In the PC12 model transfected with the cDNA under the control of the CMV promoter, expression of *pcp4* brings protection against induced apoptosis (staurosporine, UV) and regulates activation of Ca2+-CaM targets namely inhibition of nNOS activity and modulation of CaMKII calcium-independent activity [Erhardt et al 2000; Johanson et al 2000]. Moreover, PCP4 expression at the transcript or protein level is reduced in the neurodegenerative Huntington disease and its murine model [Utal et al 1998; Luthi-Carter et al 2002]. These studies have suggested that PCP4 may act as a neuroprotector in the brain.

In order to understand the possible consequences of PCP4 overexpression in trisomy 21, we have constructed cellular models with one additional copy of the gene. One of the chosen model is the human neuroblastoma SH-SY5Y in which differentiation may be induced by retinoic acid (RA). SH-SY5Y were transfected with a clone containing (1) the mouse *pcp4* gene and 5' and 3'regions which may bear regulatory elements but no other gene, (2) the PAC vector with a neomycin-resistant gene for selection after transfection. Stable tranfectants were compared with the naive SH-SY5Y. RA treatment was performed on SH-SY5Y, a neomycin-resistant clone obtained during the selection of transfectants which lack the *pcp4* gene (neoSH-SY5Y) and a clone containing one copy of the entire *pcp4* gene (P04:1). Treatment with RA induced expression of human PCP4 in SH-SY5Y at the transcript and protein level (data not shown) and this expression increased during the RA treatment (figure 5).

The same treatment induces also the expression of the murine *pcp4* gene in P04:1 (data not shown). The presence of protein markers which are known to be early neuronal (beta3-tubulin) and late neuronal polarity (tau and MAP-2) markers were analyzed by immunocytochemistry to follow the differentiation process of the cells in culture [Encinas et al 2000]. They showed that in these experimental conditions SH-SY5Y, neoSH-SY5Y and P04:1 differentiate into neurons. Neurites extended during the 14 days treatment and the different cell types were compared at 7 and 14 days of treatment. SH-SY5Y and the neoSH-SY5Y clone did not differ in their neurite extension at 7 and 14 days of treatment while the P04:1 clone containing the murine *pcp4* gene showed larger neurites at 7 and 14 days of treatment compared to the two other cells (figures 6 and 7). Percentage of growth between 7 and 14 days were identical for the three cell types indicating that the additional copy of PCP4 did not result in a different speed of neurite extension. Thus, the presence of three copies of PCP4 in the cells preferentially induced a more rapid maturation of the cells leading to an earlier differentiated phenotype of SH-SY5Y.

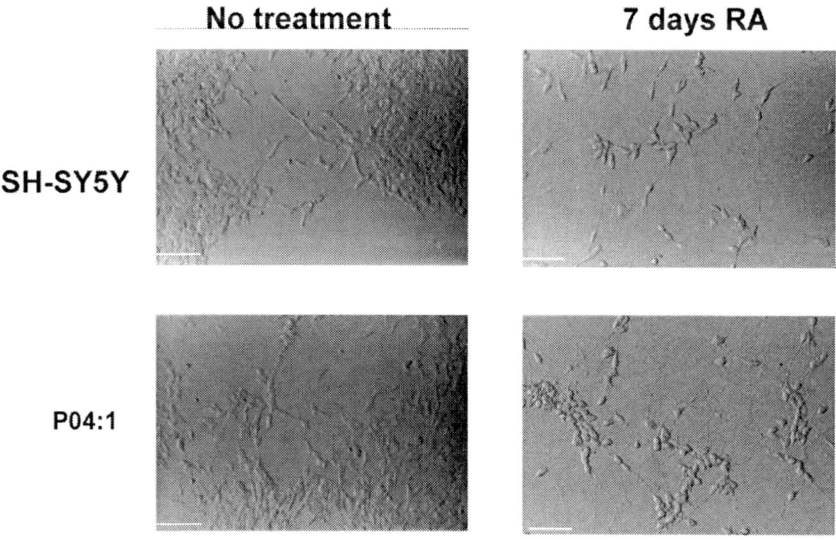

Figure 6. Morphology of cells in normal culture conditions and after 7 days of retinoic acid treatment. For the RA-induced differentiation, cells were plated onto BD-Biocoat collagen type I culture slides at a density of 10 000cells/cm2. Retinoic acid (10µM) was added the day after [as in Encinas et al 2000]. SH-SY5Y cells and P04:1 (clone transfected with the PAC clone containing the murine *pcp4* gene). Note the more numerous and larger neurites in P04:1.

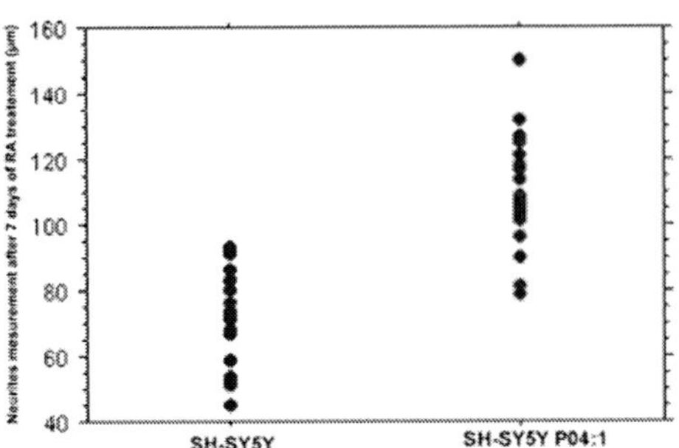

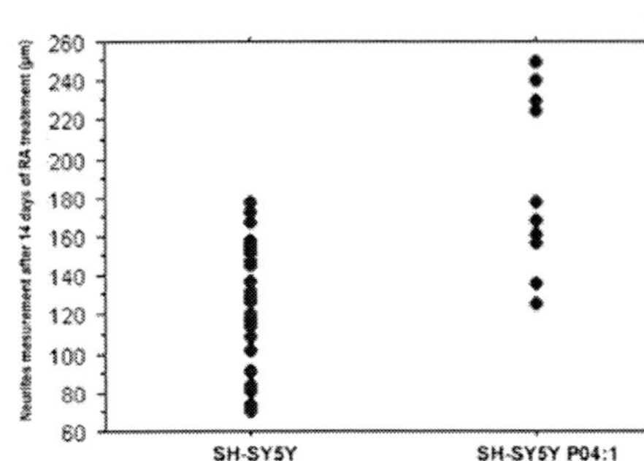

Figure 7. Measurements of neurites in the SH-SY5Y and P04:1 during RA-induced differentation at 7 and 14 days of treatment.

Expression of PCP4 during RA-induced neuron differentiation has been also shown in the human NTERA2 model [Przyborski et al 2003]. In this model, gene expression was analyzed by microarrays on NTERA2-derived neurons at 28 days in culture and showed expression of several neuronal genes including PCP4. In our experiences, we looked for expression of PCP4 earlier and we could follow its progression during the neuronal differentiation process. Moreover in the SH-SY5Y, the phenotype induced by an overexpression of PCP4 suggest that Ca2+-CaM targets, like CaMKII which is known to play a role in neurite extension [Borodinsky et al 2002], may be involved. Overexpression of PCP4 at the protein level in changing the amount of regulators of Ca2+-CaM function may accelerate the Ca2+ binding to CaM and thus the activation of Ca2+-CaM targets [Putkey et al 2005] required in the differentiation process [Gold et al 2003].

From these experiments we keep in mind that PCP4 is involved in the differentiation of neural cells and particularly of neuroblasts. Its over-expression is associated with a more rapid maturation and leads to an earlier differentiated phenotype in the NB cell line SH-SY-5Y.

Personal Data: 3 Trisomic 21 Fibroblast Extra Cellular Matrix Inhibits the Growth of Neuroblastoma Cell Lines

A body of evidence favors tumor cells microenvironment [Kenny and Bissel 2003] as a key regulator of invasion and metastasis [De Wever and Mareel 2003]. The particular distribution of neoplasms in children and adults with DS led us to the observation that neoplasms which are over-represented in this condition such as leukaemia, sarcomas, retinoblastoma and lymphoma have a poorly developed stroma, whereas tumors which are rare in DS, but frequent in the general population, such as carcinomas of the breast, colon, bronchus, prostate and skin have a well developed stroma [Satgé et al 1998a, Hasle et al 2000, Satgé et al 2003b, Patja et al 2006]. In this regards, it has been shown that i) stromal fibroblasts play an active role in early cancer development [Bhowmick et al 2004], ii) fibroblasts picked-up from normal tissues of patients with hereditary predisposition to cancer exhibit a modified phenotype that favors tumor development [Tlsty et al 2001]. On the other hand, various studies have revealed differences in the extracellular matrix composition in persons with DS, particularly of type 1, 2, 5 and 6 collagens [von Kaisenberg et al 1998], of hyaluronan [Raio et al 2005] and of matrix metalloproteinase 2 [Komatsu et al 2001]. It was thus interesting to evaluate the effect of trisomy 21 fibroblasts extracellular matrix (T21 FECM) on the growth of neoplasms which have an abundant stroma. The breast cancer cell line MDA-MB431 cultured onto an extracellular matrix (ECM) elaborated by trisomic 21 fibroblasts compared to euploid fibroblasts [Bénard et al 2005] elicited a significant growth inhibition. This interesting result prompted us to test the effect of such T21 FECM (Figure 8) on human NB cells.

In that aim we challenged, for their proliferative ability onto the T21 FECM, neuroblastoma cell lines which differ with regards to their malignant potential *in vitro* and *in vivo*: MYCN-nonamplified SK-N-SH cells, weakly MYCN-amplified SK-N-As cells, and highly MYCN-amplified IGR-N-91 able to disseminate in nude mice from subcutaneous xenograft. The T21 FECM and euploid fibroblast ECM were obtained from cultures of euploid and trisomic 21 fibroblasts that reached confluence. Thereafter, Fibroblasts were lysed by osmotic shock and preparation was extensively washed. Initially 100 000 NB cells from the three cell lines were plated on euploid fibroblasts ECM and T21 FECM. Neuroblastoma cell density measurement at 3 days post seeding, on T21 FECM as compared to euploid fibroblasts ECM, showed a significant (more than 30%) reduction in SK-N-SH and SK-N-As but not in IGR-N-91. However differences in NB cells differentiation were not observed. Although preliminary, these data strongly suggest that T21 FECM exerts, by itself and independently from factors secreted by trisomic 21 stroma cells, a growth inhibitory effect on neuroblasts of moderate malignancy but not those of high aggressiveness.

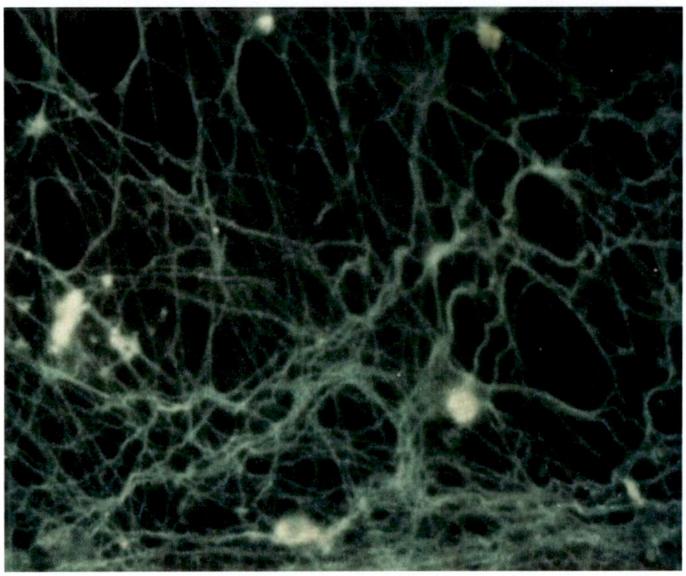

Figure 8. Network structure of DS fibroblast extracellular matrix distinguished by an anti-vimentin antibody.

A Protective Effect of Neural Cell Differentiation and Extra Cellular Medium?

The review of the literature and the epidemiological study presented [Satgé et al 1998b] clearly show that infants and children with DS are protected against NB. This protection is a beneficial consequence of the constitutional genetic imbalance due to the supernumerary chromosome 21. Thus, a search of the protective mechanism(s) must deal with genes which are triplicated in persons with DS.

The review of the currently known genes on chromosome 21 expressed in neural cells and playing a role in apoptosis, cell adhesion, cell proliferation, cell differentiation and angiogenesis shows that, due to numerous interactions, it is not possible to predict how their increased expression could affect these processes and favor or inhibit neural cell carcinogenesis. This is in agreement with Gardiner's analysis concerning the MAP kinase and the Ca-calcineurin pathways where several chromosome 21 genes interact [Gardiner 2003, Ma'ayan et al 2006] : it is not possible with the numerous experimental data to predict the final phenotypical result. However, a closer look at the review indicates that many genes directly or indirectly favor the process of neural cell maturation. First, APP, S100B and TIAM1 genes have a strong differentiating action. Furthermore, and as we already noted, enhanced cell adhesion promotes neurite outgrowth, the clearest morphological feature of neural cell differentiation. Similarly, cycle cell inhibition is a prerequisite condition for cell differentiation. Apoptosis alone cannot explain the importantly reduced frequency of NB in DS. First, because the remaining living cells which escaped apoptosis could as well become malignant, but they do not. Second, because the protection is very strong. Indeed, it is estimated that the worldly population of persons with DS is around 6,000 000. Since NB occurs 1 every 7,000 births we should expected between 800 and 900 cases in young children currently. In fact, only five cases have been reported so far since more than a century. Similarly, we do not think that inhibition of tumor-related angiogenesis can alone explain the importantly reduced number of NB in DS. Angiogenesis takes place when tumoral tissue is already built. We consider that the antineoplastic effect of DS against NB is effective very early at the first steps of oncogenesis. The extreme rarity of *in situ* NB as well as the earliest visible aspect of the tumor in fetuses, neonates and infants with DS form a strong body of argument for that.

Our preliminary experiments using S100B protein, PCP4 gene and the extracellular matrix produced by trisomic 21 fibroblasts provide additional data favoring the importance of the phenomenon of differentiation and underline the role of the extracellular medium. The ten fold reduced volume of IGR-N-91 cell line xenografts in mice which received a low dose of S100B protein in their flank, and the lack of tumor development in two of the five mice which received a high dose of S100B protein indicate that S100B protein alone may exert *in vivo* a strong inhibition of tumor proliferation. We think that S100B protein could play an important role as a powerful differentiating agent, possibly in collaboration with the interferon system. Indeed, Interferon gamma and Interferon alpha are particularly effective in tumor growth inhibition when associated with differentiating agents such as retinoic acid, valproic acid and nerve growth factor, at least in cell lines LAN-5, GI-LI-N, UKF-NB-2, UKF-NB-3 and SH-SY5Y

[Cornaglia-Ferraris et al 1992, Ridge et al 1996, Michaelis et al 2004]. We do think that other genes on chromosome 21 strengthen the differentiation pressure on neuroblasts. One of these genes, as shown for the first time in our experiments, is PCP4. The observation that one additional copy of the PCP4 gene in SH-SY5Y NB cell line produced a more rapid RA-induced differentiation leading to an earlier differentiated phenotype appears very important in the context of DS. It could indicate that this gene, when over-expressed in trisomic 21 neural cells, could lead to an earlier state of differentiation which makes the neuroblastic tissue less sensitive to neoplastic transformation.

Another point of our experiments deserving comments is the role of the extracellular medium and the role of non-tumoral cells in tumor-cell growth and differentiation. The extracellular matrix produced by trisomic 21 fibroblasts and which is different from the extracellular matrix of euploid cells [Bénard et al 2005] inhibited the growth and induced differentiation of the NB cell lines SH-SY5Y and SK-N-AS. Additionally, S100B protein which induces growth arrest and NB differentiation [Kligman and Hsieh 1987, Winningham-Major et al 1989] is not synthetized by neuroblasts, but is a main secretion product of Schwann cells and of sustentacular cells [Zimmer et al 1995]. Since Schwann cell-condition medium promotes NB differentiation [Kwiatkowski et al 1998], we wonder whether S100B protein could not be one of the important soluble agents supporting extensive neurite outgrowth. From this data we must conclude that the protection of persons with DS against NB is not only due to the over-expression of genes in neuroblasts. It is also related to the over-expression of genes in non-neural cells, at least Schwann cells, sustentacular cells in the adrenal medulla, and fibroblasts.

As NB arise from embryonal cells of the sympathetic nervous system and seem to recapitulate the development of sympathetic tissue, it is considered that the origin of neuroblastic tumors resides as a block in the process of differentiation [Israel 1993, Mora and Gerald 2004, Edsjo et al 2006]. The degree of sympathetic neuronal tissue-cell differentiation influences the patient outcome. Furthermore, treatment induced-maturation to a benign tumor has been documented [Israel 1993, Edsjo et al 2006].

In this context, it is interesting to note that no delay in neural cell maturation has been found in the nervous system of children with DS [Brooksbank et al 1989]. On the contrary, an immuno-histochemical study has shown greater neurofilament expression indicating precocious maturation [Plioplys 1987]. Furthermore, an evaluation of the cell columns development in various areas of the brain of children with DS has revealed an accelerated maturation of neural cells [Buxhoevedenn et al 2002, Buxhoeveden and Casanova 2004]. Moreover increase in arboritic dendritisation is observed in infantile DS brain, while later in development this feature is reversed [Becker et al 1991]. We believe that the reduced cellularity and hypoplasia of adrenal medulla in children with DS could as well be a consequence of precocious maturation. These observations fit well with our evaluation that over-expressed genes of chromosome 21 seem to favor neural cell over-maturation. This could be particularly true for S100B protein [Mito and Becker 1993]. Our finding that over-expression of PCP4 favors precocious maturation of neural cells in NB cell lines is in complete agreement with these observations, though the mechanism through which this modulator of Ca2+/calmodulin acts is not yet known.

This concept of increased resistance to neoplastic transformation of mature or over-mature neural cells is strengthened by an observation on testicular germ cell tissue in DS. Indeed, an analysis of the development of testicular germ cells has demonstrated a delay in maturation in fetuses with trisomy 21 [Cools et al 2006]. This could be linked to the important increased risk for testicular cancer in men with DS [Satgé et al 1997, Dieckman et al 1997]. Thus, we hypothetize that anomalies of tissue maturation in various organs play a great part in carcinogenesis (favoring neoplasms or protecting against neoplasms) for non-epithelial tumors in DS. We do not exclude that this could also be applied to persons without DS.

Conclusion

Neuroblastoma remains a highly malignant neoplasm, particularly in children older than one year, despite huge therapeutic efforts of clinical teams and of research teams, worldwide and past decades. In this context, the fact that a condition such as DS strongly protects against neuroblastic tumors is of major importance. It shows that the human body may be modified to become very resistant not only to NB, but also to other neural tumors in the central nervous system, due to constitutional genetic modification. Although these modifications are viable, the condition is responsible for important health impairments, intellectual disability being the worst. What should be investigated is, not to exactly reproduce the DS phenotype in an euploid tissue, but to avail the mechanism (or the mechanisms) which protect against neoplastic transformation in Trisomy 21 neural tissues. In other words, to find which modified subcellular compartments and which modified biochemical pathways lead to a tissue which does not allow an escape from normal growth control.

The challenge is considerable. We are not dealing with a genetic disease due to the dysregulation of one gene, however numerous are its targets and however complex its regulation. Instead, we are facing a biological condition where 300 genes or more are over-expressed, theoretically at a rate of 150%. In this context, taking into account the reduced neural cell density in DS, we have hypothetized that the protection against neuroblastoma could result from an earlier and higher pressure of differentiation. Our preliminary experiments with the PCP4 gene, S100B protein and the ECM produced by trisomic 21 fibroblasts point to the role of genes that favors neural differentiation and to the role of extracellular medium. We do not exclude the possible effect of other genes of chromosome 21 acting on other biological processes, and particularly the coincident additive effect of several genes. However, we are strongly convinced that the most important protective process is acting very early on the first events of neoplastic transformation. Therefore, we think that the knowledge of the mechanism responsible for NB protection in persons with DS could not only help to treat NB, but could also provide clues to prevent NB development in children in the general population.

Acknowledgments

The works on PCP4 gene and extra cellular matrix reported in this chapter have been supported by grants from the *Fondation Jérôme Lejeune* to N. Créau and to J. Bénard. R. Aflalo-Rattenbach was supported by the *European Community Grant 2001 – QLRT* – 00816. A grant from the *Ligue contre le Cancer division de la Corrèze* supported the epidemiological study on neuroblastoma in Down syndrome. A grant of ARAME (*Association Régionale d'Action Médicale et sociale en faveur d'Enfants atteints d'affections malignes*) supported the study on the effect of S100B protein on xenografted mice. Grants from the *Fondation Jérôme Lejeune* to D. Satgé supported the study of distribution of neoplasms in Down syndrome. We are very grateful for these supports.

Christiane Satgé is acknowledged for skill secretarial assistance.

References

Abe M, Sato Y. cDNA microarray analysis of the gene expression profile of VEGF-activated human umbilical vein endothelial cells. *Angiogenesis* 2001;4:289-98

Airoldi I, Meazza R, Croce M, Di Carlo E, Piazza T, Cocco C, D'Antuono T, Pistoia V, Ferrini S, Corrias MV. Low-dose interferon-gamma-producing human neuroblastoma cells show reduced proliferation and delayed tumorigenicity. *Br. J. Cancer* 2004; 90:2210-8

Al-Hermi BE, Thorner PS, Arbus GS. Acute plasmacytic interstitial nephritis in a child with Down syndrome. *Pediatr. Nephrol.* 1999;13:333-5

Allinquant B, Hantraye P, Mailleux P, Moya K, Bouillot C, Prochiantz A. Downregulation of amyloid precursor protein inhibits neurite outgrowth in vitro. *J. Cell Biol.* 1995;128:919-27

Allore RJ, Friend WC, O'Hanlon D, Neilson KM, Baumal R, Dunn RJ, Marks A. Cloning and expression of the human S100 beta gene. *J. Biol. Chem.* 1990;265:15537-43

Ando K, Oishi M, Takeda S, Iijima K, Isohara T, Nairn AC, Kirino Y, Greengard P, Suzuki T. Role of phosphorylation of Alzheimer's amyloid precursor protein during neuronal differentiation. *J. Neurosci.* 1999;19:4421-7

Barger GR, Douglas JG Kupski WJ, Sloan AE, Zak IT. Medulloblastoma. In: Berger MS and Prados MD (Eds). Textbook of Neuro-Oncology. Philadelphia: Elsevier Saunders; 2005;pp253-4

Barlow GM, Lyons GE, Richardson JA, Sarnat HB, Korenberg JR. DSCAM: an endogenous promoter drives expression in the developing CNS and neural crest. *Biochem. Biophys. Res. Commun.* 2002;299:1

Becker L, Mito T, Takashima S, Onodera K. Growth and development of the brain in Down syndrome. *Prog. Clin. Biol. Res.*1991;373:133-152

Bénard J, Beron-Gaillard N, Satge D. Down's syndrome protects against breast cancer: is a constitutional cell microenvironment the key? *Int. J. Cancer* 2005;113:168-70

Benda CE. Endocrine aspects of mongolism. *J. Clin. Endocrinol.* 1942;2:737-48

Benda CE. The suprarenal glands. In: Benda CE (Ed). The child with mongolism. New York: *Grune and Stratton;* 1960;pp131-9

Bhowmick NA, Neilson EG, Moses HL. Stromal fibroblasts in cancer initiation and progression. *Nature* 2004;432:332-7

Biedler JL. Helson L, Spengler BA. Morphology and growth, tumorigenicity, and cytogenetics of human neuroblastoma cells in continuous culture. *Cancer Res.* 1973; 33: 2643-52

Biedler JL, Spengler BA. A novel chromosome abnormality in human neuroblastoma and antifolate-resistant chinese hamster cell lines in culture. *J. Natl. Cancer Inst.* 1976; 57: 683-9

Boker LK, Merrick J. Cancer incidence in persons with Down syndrome in Israel. *Downs Syndr. Res. Pract.* 2002;8:31-6

Borodinsky LN, Coso OA, Fiszman ML. Contribution of Ca2+ calmodulin-dependent protein kinase II and mitogen-activated protein kinase kinase to neural activity-induced neurite outgrowth and survival of cerebellar granule cells. *J. Neurochem.* 2002; 80:1062-70

Breen KC, Bruce M, Anderton BH. Beta amyloid precursor protein mediates neuronal cell-cell and cell-surface adhesion. *J. Neurosci. Res.* 1991;28:90-100

Brooksbank BW, Walker D, Balazs R, Jorgensen OS. Neuronal maturation in the foetal brain in Down's syndrome. *Early Hum. Dev.* 1989;18:237-46

Busciglio J, Yankner BA. Apoptosis and increased generation of reactive oxygen species in Down's syndrome neurons in vitro. *Nature* 1995;378:776-9

Buxhoeveden D, Fobbs A, Roy E, Casanova M. Quantitative comparison of radial cell columns in children with Down's syndrome and controls. *J. Intellect. Disabil. Res.* 2002; 46: 76-81

Buxhoeveden D, Casanova MF. Accelerated maturation in brains of patients with Down syndrome. *J. Intellect. Disabil. Res.* 2004;48:704-5

Cabin DE, Gardiner K, Reeves RH. Molecular genetic characterization and comparative mapping of the human PCP4 gene. *Somat. Cell Mol. Genet.* 1996;22:167-75

Casanova MF, Walker LC, Whitehouse PJ, Price DL. Abnormalities of the nucleus basalis in Down's syndrome. *Ann. Neurol.* 1985;18:310-3

Ceballos-Picot I, Nicole A, Briand P, Grimber G, Delacourte A, Defossez A, Javoy-Agid F, Lafon M, Blouin JL, Sinet PM. Neuronal-specific expression of human copper-zinc superoxide dismutase gene in transgenic mice: animal model of gene dosage effects in Down's syndrome. *Brain Res.* 1991;552:198-214

Chen SL, Orr HT. Sequence of a murine cDNA, pcp-4, that encodes the homolog of the rat brain-specific antigen PEP-19. *Nucleic Acids Res.* 1990;18:1304

Cohen WI. Health car guidelines for individuals with Down syndrome. *Down Syndrome Quaterly* 1999;4:1-16

Cools M, Honecker F, Stoop H, Veltman JD, de Krijger RR, Steyerberg E, Wolffenbuttel KP, Bokemeyer C, Lau YF, Drop SL, Looijenga LH. Maturation delay of germ cells in fetuses with trisomy 21 results in increased risk for the development of testicular germ cell tumors. *Hum. Pathol.* 2006;37:101-11

Cooper MJ, Hutchins GM, Israel MA. Histogenesis of the human adrenal medulla. An evaluation of the ontogeny of chromaffin and nonchromaffin lineages. *Am. J. Pathol.* 1990; 137:605-15

Cornaglia-Ferraris P, Mariottini GL, Ponzoni M. Gamma-interferon and retinoic acid synergize in inhibiting the growth of human neuroblastoma cells in nude mice. *Cancer Lett.* 1992;61:215-20

de Haan JB, Cristiano F, Iannello R, Bladier C, Kelner MJ, Kola I. Elevation in the ratio of Cu/Zn-superoxide dismutase to glutathione peroxidase activity induces features of cellular senescence and this effect is mediated by hydrogen peroxide. *Hum. Mol. Genet.* 1996; 5: 283-92

Delfini C. Contributo allo studio del mongolismo. *Rev Speriment Pediatr. Med. Legale.* 1932; 56:162-217

De Wever O, Mareel M. Role of tissue stroma in cancer cell invasion. *J. Pathol.* 2003; 200: 429-47

Dickerson JB, Morgan MA, Mishra A, Slaughter CA, Morgan JI, Zheng J. The influence of phosphorylation on the activity and structure of the neuronal IQ motif protein, PEP-19. *Brain Res.* 2006;1092:16-27

Dieckmann KP, Rube C, Henke RP. Association of Down's syndrome and testicular cancer. *J. Urol.* 1997;157:1701-4

Dixon N, Kishnani PS, Zimmerman S. Clinical manifestations of hematologic and oncologic disorders in patients with Down syndrome. *Am. J. Med. Genet. C Semin. Med. Genet.* 2006; 142:149-57

Donato R. Functional roles of S100 proteins, calcium-binding proteins of the EF-hand type. *Biochim. Biophys. Acta.* 1999;1450:191-231

Donato R. Intracellular and extracellular roles of S100 proteins. *Microsc. Res. Tech.* 2003; 60:540-51

Eberhard Y, Eterradossi J, Therminarias A. Biochemical changes and catecholamine responses in Down's syndrome adolescents in relation to incremental maximal exercise. *J. Ment. Defic. Res.* 1991;35 :140-6

Edsjo A, Holmquist L, Pahlman S. Neuroblastoma as an experimental model for neuronal differentiation and hypoxia-induced tumor cell dedifferentiation. *Semin. Cancer Biol.* 2006 (in press)

El-Ghissassi F, Valsesia-Wittmann S, Falette N, Duriez C, Walden PD, Puisieux A. BTG2(TIS21/PC3) induces neuronal differentiation and prevents apoptosis of terminally differentiated PC12 cells. *Oncogene* 2002;21:6772-78

Encinas M, Iglesias M, Liu Y, Wang H, Muhaisen A, Cena V, Gallego C, Comella JX. Sequential treatment of SH-SY5Y cells with retinoic acid and brain-derived neurotrophic factor gives rise to fully differentiated, neurotrophic factor-dependent, human neuron-like cells. *J. Neurochem.* 2000;75:991-1003

Epstein CJ. Specificity versus nonspecificity in the pathogenesis of aneuploid phenotypes. *Am. J. Med. Genet.* 1988 ;29:161-5

Epstein CJ. The consequences of chromosome imbalance. *Am. J. Med. Genet. Suppl.* 1990; 7: 31-7

Epstein CJ. Down syndrome (trisomy 21). In: Scriver CR, Beaudet AL, Sly WS, Valle D. (Eds). *The metabolic and molecular bases of inherited diseases.* New York: McGraw-hill; 2001;pp1223-57

Erhardt JA, Legos JJ, Johanson RA, Slemmon JR, Wang X. Expression of PEP-19 inhibits apoptosis in PC12 cells. *Neuroreport* 2000;11:3719-23

Fabia J, Drolette M. Malformations and leukemia in children with Down's syndrome. *Pediatrics* 1970;45:60-70

Fano G, Mariggio MA, Angelella P, Nicoletti I, Antonica A, Fulle S, Calissano P. The S-100 protein causes an increase of intracellular calcium and death of PC12 cells. *Neuroscience* 1993; 53:919-25

Feingold M, Gheradi GJ, Simons C. Familial neuroblastoma and trisomy 13. *Am. J. Dis. Child* 1971;121:451

Fernhall B, Otterstetter M. Attenuated responses to sympathoexcitation in individuals with Down syndrome. *J. Appl. Physiol.* 2003;94:2158-65

Ferrandis E, Da Silva J, Riou G, Benard I. Coactivation of the MDR1 and MYCN genes in human neuroblastoma cells during the metastatic process in the nude mouse. *Cancer Res.* 1994; 54:2256-61

Fitzpatrick DR. Transcriptional consequences of autosomal trisomy: primary gene dosage with complex downstream effects. *Trends Genet.* 2005;21:249-53

Foos G, Garcia-Ramirez JJ, Galang CK, Hauser CA. Elevated expression of Ets2 or distinct portions of Ets2 can reverse Ras-mediated cellular transformation. *J. Biol. Chem.* 1998; 273: 18871-80

Foulkes WD, Buu PN, Filiatrault D, Leclerc JM, Narod SA. Excess of congenital abnormalities in French-Canadian children with neuroblastoma: a case series study from Montreal. *Med. Pediatr. Oncol.* 1997;29:272-9

Fuentes JJ, Genesca L, Kingsbury TJ, Cunningham KW, Perez-Riba M, Estivill X, de la Luna S. DSCR1, overexpressed in Down syndrome, is an inhibitor of calcineurin-mediated signaling pathways. *Hum. Mol. Genet.* 2000;9:1681-90

Gandolfi A, Horoupian DS, De Teresa RM. Pathology of the auditory system in autosomal trisomies with morphometric and quantitative study of the ventral cochlear nucleus. *J. Neurol. Sci.* 1981;51:43-50

Gardiner K. Predicting pathway perturbations in Down syndrome. *J. Neural. Transm. Suppl.* 2003; 67:21-37

Gardiner K, Davisson MT, Pritchard M, Patterson D, Groner Y, Crnic LS, Antonarakis S, Mobley W. Report on the 'Expert Workshop on the Biology of Chromosome 21: towards gene-phenotype correlations in Down syndrome', held June 11-14, 2004, Washington D.C. *Cytogenet. Genome Res.* 2005;108:269-77

Geraci AP, de Csepel J, Shlasko E, Wallace SA. Ganglioneuroblastoma and ganglioneuroma in association with neurofibromatosis type I: report of three cases. *J. Child Neurol.* 1998; 13: 356-8

Gerendasy D. Homeostatic tuning of Ca2+ signal transduction by members of the calpacitin protein family. *J. Neurosci. Res.* 1999;58:107-19

Gold DA, Baek SH, Schork NJ, Rose DW, Larsen DD, Sachs BD, Rosenfeld MG, Hamilton BA RORalpha coordinates reciprocal signaling in cerebellar development through sonic hedgehog and calcium-dependent pathways. *Neuron* 2003;40:1119-31

Gordon MB. Morphological changes in the endocrine glands in Mongolian idiocy with report of two cases. *Endocrinology* 1930;14:1-6

Hachitanda Y, Nakagawara A, Nagoshi M, Tsuneyoshi M. Prognostic value of *N-myc* oncogene amplification and S-100 protein positivity in children with neuroblastic tumors. *Acta Pathol. Jpn.* 1992;42:639-44

Harimaya K, Oda Y, Matsuda S, Tanaka K, Chuman H, Iwamoto Y. Primitive neuroectodermal tumor and extraskeletal Ewing sarcoma arising primarily around the spinal column: report of four cases and a review of the literature. *Spine* 2003;28:E408-12

Hasle H, Clemmensen IH, Mikkelsen M. Risks of leukaemia and solid tumours in individuals with Down's syndrome. *Lancet* 2000;355:165-9

Hattori M, Fujiyama A, Taylor TD, Watanabe H, Yada T, Park HS, Toyoda A, Ishii K, Totoki Y, Choi DK, Groner Y, Soeda E, Ohki M, Takagi T, Sakaki Y, Taudien S, Blechschmidt K, Polley A, Menzel U, Delabar J, Kumpf K, Lehmann R, Patterson D, Reichwald K, Rump A, Schillhabel M, Schudy A, Zimmermann W, Rosenthal A, Kudoh J, Schibuya K, Kawasaki K, Asakawa

S, Shintani A, Sasaki T, Nagamine K, Mitsuyama S, Antonarakis SE, Minoshima S, Shimizu N, Nordsiek G, Hornischer K, Brant P, Scharfe M, Schon O, Desario A, Reichelt J, Kauer G, Blocker H, Ramser J, Beck A, Klages S, Hennig S, Riesselmann L, Dagand E, Haaf T, Wehrmeyer S, Borzym K, Gardiner K, Nizetic D, Francis F, Lehrach H, Reinhardt R, Yaspo ML; Chromosome 21 mapping and sequencing consortium. The DNA sequence of human chromosome 21. *Nature* 2000;405:311-9

Hosoi H, Sawada T, Nakajima T, Kuroda H, Saida T, Sugimoto T, Tokiwa K, Ogita S. A case of mosaic Down's syndrome concomitant with ganglioneuroma. *J. Pediatr. Surg.* 1989; 24:210-1

Hu J, Ferreira A, van Eldik LJ. S100β induces neuronal cell death through nitric oxide release from astrocytes. *J. Neurochem.* 1997;69:2294-301

Huttunen HJ, Kuja-Panula J, Sorci G, Agneletti AL, Donato R, Rauvala H. Coregulation of neurite outgrowth and cell survival by amphoterin and S100 proteins through receptor for advanced glycation end products (RAGE) activation. *J. Biol. Chem.* 2000;275:40096-105

Isaacs H Jr. Neuroblastoma in situ. In: Isaacs H Jr (Ed). Tumors of the fetus and newborn. Philadelphia: WB Saunders; 1997;p145

Israel MA. Disordered differentiation as a target for novel approaches to the treatment of neuroblastoma. *Cancer* 1993;71:3310-3

Iwanaga T, Fujita T. Sustentacular cells in the fetal human adrenal medulla are immunoreactive with antibodies to brain S-100 protein. *Cell Tissue Res.* 1984;236:733-5

Johanson RA, Sarau HM, Foley JJ, Slemmon JR. Calmodulin-binding peptide PEP-19 modulates activation of calmodulin kinase II In situ. *J. Neurosci.* 2000;20:2860-6

Joshi VV, Balarezo F, Hicks MJ, Mierau GW, Tsongalis GJ. Approach to small round cell tumors of childhood. *Pathology case Reviews* 2000;5:26-41

Kenny PA, Bissell MJ. Tumor reversion: correction of malignant behavior by microenvironmental cues. *Int. J. Cancer* 2003;107:688-95

Kissane JM. Introdution, Embryonal tumors. *Semin. Diagn. Pathol.* 1994;11:83-4

Kligman D, Hsieh LS. Neurite extension factor induces rapid morphological differentiation of mouse neuroblastoma cells in defined medium. *Dev. Brain Res.* 1987;33:296-300

Komatsu T, Kubota E, Sakai N. Enhancement of matrix metalloproteinase (MMP)-2 activity in gingival tissue and cultured fibroblasts from Down's syndrome patients. *Oral Dis.* 2001; 7:47-55

Korenberg JR, Chen XN, Schipper R, Sun Z, Gonsky R, Gerwehr S, Carpenter N, Daumer C, Dignan P, Disteche C, et al. Down syndrome phenotypes: the consequences of chromosomal imbalance. *Proc. Natl. Acad. Sci. USA.* 1994;91:4997-5001

Koyama T, Kanadani T, Tanaka M, Nakahara S, Yamadori I. A case of Down's syndrome associated with progressive extradural neuroblastoma. *Pediatr. Surg. Int.* 1999;15:373-5

Kramer S, Ward E, Meadows AT, Malone KE. Medical and drug risk factors associated with neuroblastoma: a case-control study. *J. Natl. Cancer Inst.* 1987;78:797-804

Kreiner E. Weight and shape of the human adrenal medulla in various age groups. *Virchows Arch. A Pathol. Anat. Histol.* 1982;397:7-15

Kuroiwa M, Takeuchi T, Lee JH, Yoshizawa J, Hirato J, Kaneko S, Choi SH, Suzuki N, Ikeda H, Tsuchida Y. Continuous versus intermittent administration of human endostatin in xenografted human neuroblastoma. *J. Pediatr. Surg.* 2003;38:1499-505

Kwiatkowski JL, Rutkowski JL, Yamashiro DJ, Tennekoon GI, Brodeur GM. Schwann cell-conditioned medium promotes neuroblastoma survival and differentiation. *Cancer Res.* 1998; 58:4602-6

Lake CR, Ziegler MG, Coleman M, Kopin IJ. Evaluation of the sympathetic nervous system in trisomy-21 (Down's syndrome). *J. Psychiatr. Res.* 1979;15(1):1-6

Lange P. Beitrag zur patologischen Anatomie des Mongolismus. *Monatsschr. Kinderheilkd.* 1906; 5:233-43

Lejeune J, Gautier M, Turpin R. Study of somatic chromosomes from 9 mongoloid children. *C R Acad. Sci.* 1959;248:1721-2

Lhermitte J. Sloboziano H., Radovici A. Contribution à l'étude anatomique de l'idiotie mongolienne. *Bull. Soc. Pediat. Paris.* 1921;19:187-96

Luthi-Carter R, Hanson SA, Strand AD, Bergstrom DA, Chun W, Peters NL, Woods AM, Chan EY, Kooperberg C, Krainc D, Young AB, Tapscott SJ, Olson JM. Dysregulation of gene expression in the R6/2 model of polyglutamine disease: parallel changes in muscle and brain. *Hum. Mol. Genet.* 2002;11:1911-26

Ma'ayan A, Gardiner K, Iyengar R. The cognitive phenotype of Down syndrome: insights from intracellular network analysis. *NeuroRx.* 2006;3:396-406

Magro G, Grasso S. Immunohistochemical identification and comparison of glial cell lineage in foetal, neonatal, adult and neoplastic human adrenal medulla. *Histochem. J.* 1997; 29: 293-9

Marcus K, Johnson M, Adam RM, O'Reilly MS, Donovan M, Atala A, Freeman MR, Soker S. Tumor cell-associated neuropilin-1 and vascular endothelial growth factor expression as determinants of tumor growth in neuroblastoma. *Neuropathology* 2005;25:178-87

Marenholz I, Heizmann CW, Fritz G. S100 proteins in mouse and man: from evolution to function and pathology (including an update of the nomenclature). *Biochem. Biophys. Res. Commun.* 2004; 322: 1111-22

Maris JM, Kyemba SM, Rebbeck TR, White PS, Sulman EP, Jensen SJ, Allen C, Biegel JA, Brodeur GM. Molecular genetic analysis of familial neuroblastoma. *Eur. J. Cancer* 1997; 33:1923-8

McSwigan JD, Hanson DR, Lubiniecki A, Heston LL, Sheppard JR. Down syndrome fibroblasts are hyperresponsive to beta-adrenergic stimulation. *Proc. Natl. Acad. Sci. USA* 1981;78:7670-3

McWilliams N.B. Neuroblastoma in infancy. In: Neuroblastoma: tumor biology and therapy. Pocheldy C (Ed). Boca Raton: CRC Press; 1990;pp229-43

Michaelis M, Suhan T, Cinatl J, Driever PH, Cinatl J Jr. Valproic acid and interferon-alpha synergistically inhibit neuroblastoma cell growth in vitro and in vivo. *Int. J. Oncol.* 2004; 25:1795-9

Michetti F, Larocca LM, Rinelli A, Lauriola L. Immunocytochemical distribution of S-100 protein in patients with Down's syndrome. *Acta Neuropathol.* 1990;80:475-8.

Miller RW, Fraumeni JF Jr, Hill JA. Neuroblastoma: epidemiologic approach to its origin. *Am. J. Dis. Child* 1968;115:253-61

Miller RW. Childhood cancer and congenital defects. A study of U.S. death certificates during the period 1960-1966. *Pediatr. Res.* 1969;3:389-97

Minami T, Horiuchi K, Miura M, Abid MR, Takabe W, Noguchi N, Kohro T, Ge X, Aburatani H, Hamakubo T, Kodama T, Aird WC. Vascular endothelial growth factor- and thrombin-induced termination factor, Down syndrome critical region-1, attenuates endothelial cell proliferation and angiogenesis. *J. Biol. Chem.* 2004;279:50537-54

Misugi K, Aoki I, Kikyo S, Sasaki Y, Tsunoda A, Nakajima T. Immunohistochemical study of neuroblastoma and related tumors with anti-S-100 protein antibody. *Pediatr. Pathol.* 1985; 3:217-26

Mito T, Becker LE. Developmental changes of S-100 protein and glial fibrillary acidic protein in the brain in Down syndrome. *Exp. Neurol.* 1993;120:170-6

Moore BW. A soluble protein characteristic of the nervous system.. *Biochem. Biophys. Res. Commun.* 1965;19:739-44

Mora J, Gerald WL. Origin of neuroblastic tumors: clues for future therapeutics. *Expert Rev. Mol. Diagn.* 2004;4:293-302

Nagoshi M, Tsuneyoshi M, Enjoji M. S-100 positive undifferentiated neuroblastomas with a special reference to the tumor stroma related to favorable prognosis. *Pathol. Res. Pract.* 1992; 188:273-83

Nakazato Y, Landing BH. Reduced number of neurons in esophageal plexus ganglia in Down syndrome: additional evidence for reduced cell number as a basic feature of the disorder. *Pediatr. Pathol.* 1986;5:55-63

Narod SA, Stiller C, Lenoir GM. An estimate of the heritable fraction of childhood cancer. *Br. J. Cancer* 1991;63:993-9

Neglia JP, Smithson WA, Gunderson P, King FL, Singher LJ, Robison LL. Prenatal and perinatal risk factors for neuroblastoma. A case-control study. *Cancer* 1988;61:2202-6

Nevin NC, Dodge JA, Allen IV. Two cases of trisomy D associated with adrenal tumours. *J. Med. Genet.* 1972;9:119-22

Nishi M, Miyake H, Takeda T, Hatae Y. Congenital malformations and childhood cancer. *Med. Pediatr. Oncol.* 2000;34:250-4

Nishiyama H, Knopfel T, Endo S, Itohara S. Glial protein S100B modulates long-term neuronal synaptic plasticity. *Proc. Natl. Acad. Sci. USA*. 2002;99:4037-42

Olshan AF, Bunin GR. Epidemiology of neuroblastoma. In: Brodeur GM, Sawada T, Tsuchida Y, Voute PA, (Eds). *Neuroblastoma*. Amsterdam. Elsevier; 2000;pp33-9

Patja K, Pukkala E, Sund R, Iivanainen M, Kaski M. Cancer incidence of persons with Down syndrome in Finland: a population-based study. *Int. J. Cancer* 2006;118:1769-72

Pearson ADJ, Pinkerton R. Neuroblastoma. In: Pinkerton R, Plowman PN, Pieters R, (Eds). Pediatric Oncology *3rd edition. London: Arnold; 2004;pp386-7*

Pennacchietti M. Contributo anatomo-patologico allo studio della idioza mongoloide. *Endocrinologia Patologia* 1935;10:148-64

Pearlson GD, Breiter SN, Aylward EH, Warren AC, Grygorcewicz M, Frangou S, Barta PE, Pulsifer MB. MRI brain changes in subjects with Down syndrome with and without dementia. *Dev. Med. Child Neurol.* 1998;40:326-34

Pine SS, Landing BH, Shankle WR. Reduced inferior olivary neuron number in early Down syndrome. *Pediatr. Pathol. Lab. Med.* 1997;17:537-45

Plioplys AV. Down's syndrome. Precocious neurofilament antigen expression. *J. Neurol. Sci.* 1987; 79:91-100

Przyborski SA, Smith S, Wood A. Transcriptional profiling of neuronal differentiation by human embryonal carcinoma stem cells in vitro. *Stem Cells* 2003;21:459-71

Putkey JA, Kleerekoper Q, Gaertner TR, Waxham MN. A new role for IQ motif proteins in regulating calmodulin function. *J. Biol. Chem.* 2003;278:49667-70

Qiu WQ, Ferreira A, Miller C, Koo EH, Selkoe DJ. Cell-surface beta-amyloid precursor protein stimulates neurite outgrowth of hippocampal neurons in an isoform-dependent manner. *J. Neurosci.* 1995;15:2157-67

Raio L, Cromi A, Ghezzi F, Passi A, Karousou E, Viola M, Vigetti D, De Luca G, Bolis P. Hyaluronan content of Wharton's jelly in healthy and Down syndrome fetuses. *Matrix Biol.* 2005;24:166-74

Ribatti D, Nico B, Pezzolo A, Vacca A, Meazza R, Cinti R, Carlini B, Parodi F, Pistoia V, Corrias MV. Angiogenesis in a human neuroblastoma xenograft model: mechanisms and inhibition by tumour-derived interferon-gamma. *Br. J. Cancer* 2006;94:1845-52

Rickert CH, Gocke H, Paulus W. Fetal ependymoma associated with Down's syndrome. *Acta Neuropathol.* 2002;103:78-81

Ridge J, Terle DA, Dragunsky E, Levenbook I. Effects of gamma-IFN and NGF on subpopulations in a human neuroblastoma cell line: flow cytometric and morphological analysis. *In Vitro Cell Dev. Biol. Anim.* 1996;32:238-48

Robinson MG, McCorquodale MM. Trisomy 18 and neurogenic neoplasia. *J. Pediatr.* 1981; 99:428-9

Rohrer T, Trachsel D, Engelcke G, Hammer J. Congenital central hypoventilation syndrome associated with Hirschsprung's disease and neuroblastoma: case of multiple neurocristopathies. *Pediatr Pulmonol.* 2002;33:71-6

Roper RJ, Reeves RH. Understanding the basis for Down syndrome phenotypes. *PLoS Genet.* 2006;2:e50

Russell BG, Kjaer I. Tooth agenesis in Down syndrome. *Am J Med Genet.* 1995;55:466-71

Sangameswaran L, Hempstead J, Morgan JI. Molecular cloning of a neuron-specific transcript and its regulation during normal and aberrant cerebellar development. *Proc. Natl. Acad. Sci. USA.* 1989;86:5651-5

Sasco AJ, Gendre I, Verbier-Naneix C, Soulier J-L, Raffi F, Satgé D, Robert E. Neonatal neuroblastoma *in utero* exposure to progestagens. *Int. J. Risk Safety Med.* 1998;11:121-8

Satgé D. A decreased incidence of neuroblastomas in Down's syndrome and overproduction of S-100 b protein. *Med. Hypotheses* 1996;46:393-9

Satgé D, Van den Berghe H. Aspects of the neoplasms observed in patients with constitutional autosomal trisomy. *Cancer Genet. Cytogenet.* 1996;87:63-70

Satgé D, Sasco AJ, Cure H, Leduc B, Sommelet D, Vekemans MJ. An excess of testicular germ cell tumors in Down's syndrome: three case reports and a review of the literature. *Cancer* 1997;80:929-35

Satgé D, Sommelet D, Geneix A, Nishi M, Malet P, Vekemans M. A tumor profile in Down syndrome. *Am. J. Med. Genet.* 1998a;78:207-16

Satgé D, Sasco AJ, Carlsen NL, Stiller CA, Rubie H, Hero B, de Bernardi B, de Kraker J, Coze C, Kogner P, Langmark F, Hakvoort-Cammel FG, Beck D, von der Weid N, Parkes S, Hartmann O, Lippens RJ, Kamps WA, Sommelet D. A lack of neuroblastoma in Down syndrome: a study from 11 European countries. *Cancer Res.* 1998b;58:448-52

Satgé D, Rubie H, Sommelet D. Paravertebral neoplasm in a child with Down syndrome (DS). *Pediatr. Surg. Int.* 2001a;17:251

Satgé D, Monteil P, Sasco AJ, Vital A, Ohgaki H, Geneix A, Malet P, Vekemans M, Rethore MO. Aspects of intracranial and spinal tumors in patients with Down syndrome and report of a rapidly progressing Grade 2 astrocytoma. *Cancer* 2001b;91:1458-66

Satgé D, Moore SW, Stiller CA, Niggli FK, Pritchard-Jones K, Bown N, Benard J, Plantaz D. Abnormal constitutional karyotypes in patients with neuroblastoma: a report of four new cases and review of 47 others in the literature. *Cancer Genet. Cytogenet.* 2003a;147:89-98

Satgé D, Sasco AJ, Chompret A, Orbach D, Mechinaud F, Lacour B, Roullet B, Martelli H, Bergeron C, Bertrand Y, Lacombe D, Perel Y, Monteil P, Nelken B, Bertozzi AI, Munzer M, Kanold J, Bernard F, Vekemans MJ, Sommelet D. A 22-year French experience with solid tumors in children with Down syndrome. *Pediatr. Hematol. Oncol.* 2003b;20:517-29

Schneid H, Vazquez MP, Vacher C, Gourmelen M, Cabrol S, Le Bouc Y. The Beckwith-Wiedemann syndrome phenotype and the risk of cancer. *Med. Pediatr. Oncol.* 1997; 28: 411-5

Selinfreund RH, Barger SW, Pledger WJ, van Eldik LJ. Neurotrophic protein S100β stimulates glial cell proliferation. *Proc. Natl. Acad. Sci. USA* 1991;88:3554-8

Shaked GM, Kummer MP, Lu DC, Galvan V, Bredesen DE, Koo EH. Abeta induces cell death by direct interaction with its cognate extracellular domain on APP (APP 597-624). *FASEB J.* 2006;20:1254-6

Shanklin DR, Sotelo-Avila C. In situ tumors in fetuses, newborns and young infants. *Biol. Neonat.* 1969;14:286-316

Shehata BM, Abramowsky CR. Alveolar capillary dysplasia in an infant with trisomy 21. *Pediatr. Dev. Pathol.* 2005;8:696-700

Sheppard JR, Schumacher W, White JG, Jakobs KH, Schultz G. The alpha adrenergic response of Down's syndrome platelets. *J. Pharmacol. Exp. Ther.* 1983;225:584-8

Shimada H, Aoyama C, Chiba T, Newton WA. Prognostic subgroups for undifferentiated neuroblastoma. *Hum. Pathol.* 1985;16:471-6

Shojaei-Brosseau T, Chompret A, Abel A, de Vathaire F, Raquin MA, Brugieres L, Feunteun J, Hartmann O, Bonaiti-Pellie C. Genetic epidemiology of neuroblastoma: a study of 426 cases at the Institut Gustave-Roussy in France. *Pediatr. Blood Cancer* 2004;42:99-105

Skog J, Mei YF, Wadell G. Human adenovirus serotypes 4p and 11p are efficiently expressed in cell lines of neural tumour origin. *J. Gen. Virol.* 2002;83:1299-309

Slemmon JR, Morgan JI, Fullerton SM, Danho W, Hilbush BS, Wengenack TM. Camstatins are peptide antagonists of calmodulin based upon a conserved structural motif in PEP-19, neurogranin, and neuromodulin. *J. Biol. Chem.* 1996;271:15911-7

Spiryda LB, Colman DR. Suppression of tumorigenicity in an aggressive cervical carcinoma induced by protein zero, a nervous system IgCAM. *J. Cell Sci.* 1998;111:3253-60

Stiller CA. Aetiology and epidemiology. In: Pinkerton R, Plowman PN, Pieters R, (Eds). Pediatric Oncology 3rd edition. London: Arnold; 2004;pp3-18

Streck CJ, Zhang Y, Miyamoto R, Zhou J, Ng CY, Nathwani AC, Davidoff AM. Restriction of neuroblastoma angiogenesis and growth by interferon-alpha/beta. *Surgery* 2004;136: 183-9

Sy WM, Edmonson JH. The development defects associated with neuroblastoma--etiologic implications. *Cancer* 1968;22:234-8

Sylvester PE. The hippocampus in Down's syndrome. *J. Ment. Defic. Res.* 1983;27:227-36

Tan YH, Schneider EL, Tischfield J, Epstein CJ, Ruddle FH. Human chromosome 21 dosage: effect on the expression of the interferon induced antiviral state. *Science* 1974;186:61-3

Tanaka M, Ohashi R, Nakamura R, Shinmura K, Kamo T, Sakai R, Sugimura H. Tiam1 mediates neurite outgrowth induced by ephrin-B1 and EphA2. *EMBO J.* 2004;23:1075-88

Tatafiore E. Ricerche anatomo-patologiche sull'encefalo e sulle ghiandole a secrezione interna di due lattanti mongoli. *Folia Medica* 1937;22:1209-36

Thiele CJ. Neuroblastoma. In: Masters JRW and Palsson B (Eds). *Human cell culture*, vol 1. Dordrecht, Great Britain. Kluwer Academic Publishers; 1999;pp21-53

Thomas S, Thiery E, Aflalo R, Vayssettes C, Verney C, Berthuy I, Creau N. PCP4 is highly expressed in ectoderm and particularly in neuroectoderm derivatives during mouse embryogenesis. *Gene Expr. Patterns* 2003;3:93-7

Tirode F, Laud-Duval K, Prieur A, Delorme B, Chaarbord P, Delattre O. Les cellules souches mésenchymateuses sont à l'origine des tumeurs d'Ewing. *Bull. Cancer* 2006;93:554

Tlsty TD, Hein PW. Know thy neighbor: stromal cells can contribute oncogenic signals. *Curr. Opin. Genet. Dev.* 2001;11:54-9

Trebo M, Klaassen R, Weitzman S. Brief report: Neuroblastoma in Down syndrome. *Med. Pediatr. Oncol.* 1999;33:125

Turkel SB, Itabashi HH. The natural history of neuroblastic cells in the fetal adrenal gland. *Am. J. Pathol.* 1974;76:225-44

Utal AK, Stopka AL, Roy M, Coleman PD. PEP-19 immunohistochemistry defines the basal ganglia and associated structures in the adult human brain, and is dramatically reduced in Huntington's disease. *Neuroscience* 1998;86:1055-63

von Kaisenberg CS, Krenn V, Ludwig M, Nicolaides KH, Brand-Saberi B. Morphological classification of nuchal skin in human fetuses with trisomy 21, 18, and 13 at 12-18 weeks and in a trisomy 16 mouse. *Anat. Embryol.* 1998;197:105-24

Winningham-Major F, Staecker JL, Barger SW, Coats S, Van Eldik LJ. Neurite extension and neuronal survival activities of recombinant S100 beta proteins that differ in the content and position of cysteine residues. *J. Cell Biol.* 1989;109:3063-71

Wolvetang EJ, Bradfield OM, Hatzistavrou T, Crack PJ, Busciglio J, Kola I, Hertzog PJ. Overexpression of the chromosome 21 transcription factor Ets2 induces neuronal apoptosis. *Neurobiol. Dis.* 2003;14:349-56

Yang Q, Rasmussen SA, Friedman JM. Mortality associated with Down's syndrome in the USA from 1983 to 1997: a population-based study. *Lancet* 2002;359:1019-25

Yoshida Y, Matsuda S, Ikematsu N, Kawamura-Tsuzuku J, Inazawa J, Umemori H, Yamamoto T. ANA, a novel member of Tob/BTG1 family, is expressed in the ventricular zone of the developing central nervous system. *Oncogene* 1998;16:2687-93

Zheng H, Koo EH. The amyloid precursor protein: beyond amyloid. *Mol. Neurodegener*. 2006;1:5

Zimmer DB, Cornwall EH, Landar A, Song W. The S100 protein family: history, function, and expression. *Brain Res. Bull.* 1995;37:417-29

Zorick TS, Mustacchi Z, Bando SY, Zatz M, Moreira-Filho CA, Olsen B, Passos-Bueno MR. High serum endostatin levels in Down syndrome: implications for improved treatment and prevention of solid tumours. *Eur. J. Hum. Genet.* 2001;9:811-4

In: Neuroblastoma Research Trends
Editors: L. H. Andre and N. E. Roux ISBN: 978-1-60456-790-8

Chapter IV

The p73 Target Genes in Human Malignant Neuroblasts are Related to Neuronal Development and Sympathetic Differentiation

***Emilie Horvilleur*[1], *David Goldschneider*[1], *Jean Bénard*[1,2], and *Sétha Douc-Rasy*[1,3]**

1. Centre National de Recherche Scientifique-Unité Mixte de Recherche 8126-Université Paris-Sud 11, Institut Gustave Roussy, 94805, Villejuif, France
2. Département de Pathologie et Biologie Médicales, Institut Gustave Roussy, 94805, Villejuif, France;
3. Université Pierre et Marie Curie, Jussieu, Paris, France

Abstract

In human neuroblastoma (NB), the wild-type (wt) p53 protein is retained in the cytoplasm of malignant neuroblasts, where it is unable to operate as a tumor suppressor in the nucleus. p73, the first homologue of the p53 gene, encodes a myriad of isoforms and variants due to alternative splicing at the NH2-or COOH-terminal regions and alternative promoter usage. Two promoters have been described so far: P1, which encodes full-length TAp73α, and the cryptic promoter P2, which is located in intron 3 and produces ΔNp73α, an N-truncated variant lacking the transactivation domain. It has been shown that TAp73α can induce tumor suppressor properties such as cell-cycle arrest and apoptosis while ΔNp73α antagonizes the pro-apoptotic p53 in sympathetic neurons upon NGF withdrawal, thus acting as a dominant negative isoform. Data from previous studies of ours indicates that overexpressed TAp73 cooperates with wtp53 to induce apoptosis with high efficiency in wtp53 NB cells but not in mutated-p53 NB cells. This prompted us to postulate that TAp73 might be a candidate for neuronal differentiation, a biological process which hallmarks NB cells and is associated with specific protein expression. To explore this possibility, we infected two human NB cell lines, SH-SY5Y and IGR-N-91, with wtp53 and mutated p53, respectively, with TAp73alpha and ΔNp73α recombinant adenoviruses. cDNA macroarray analysis with the Atlas Human Cancer 1.2 Array (Clontech) showed that: i) TAp73α transactivated the expression of a number of genes associated with development and neuronal function, including Notch1, MIC-1/GDF-15, Jagged2, $p75^{NTR}$ (NGFR), and chromogranin B in both cell lines; ii) ΔNp73α inhibited these developmental genes and repressed the S100 calcium-binding protein, known to be implicated in neuronal differentiation; iii) Wnt8A, known to be involved in development and neuronal differentiation, was only activated by TA-or ΔNp73 in SH-SY5Y cells, suggesting that transactivation in this case is not dependent on the NH2-terminal transactivation domain.

Keywords: *Neuroblastoma; p53; p73; Expression profile; Macroarray; Development; Neuronal differentiation*

Abbreviations

NB, neuroblastoma; NGF, nerve growth factor; NTR, neurotrophin receptor; EphA2, EphrinA receptor 2; BTG2, B-cell translocation gene 2; FACS, fluorescence-activated cell sorting; PLGF, placental growth factor.

1. Introduction

Neuroblastoma (NB), the most common form of pediatric solid tumor in very early childhood, originates in the neural crest and causes tumors in the adrenal medulla, the paravertebral sympathetic ganglia, and the sympathetic paraganglia [Shimada et al., 1999]. At the histological level, neuroblastic tumors encompass a spectrum of 5 major types, ranging from undifferentiated Schwannian stroma-poor neuroblastoma (NB) to fully differentiated Schwannian stroma-dominant ganglioneuroma (GN); between these 2 extremes, there are 3 composite types, which display a progressive gradient of differentiation: NB/GNB (ganglioneuroblastoma), GNB, and GNB/GN (Figure 1).

Abnormalities of the *p53* tumor suppresor gene are commonly found in over 50% of human cancers, but in NB tumors, the p53 protein is non fonctional although it is a wild-type protein. Several studies support this non mutational inactivation as a consequence of cytoplasmic sequestration and defective translocation of p53 into the nucleus [Moll, 1995]; [Ostermeyer 1996]; [Nikolaev, 2003]. The discoveries of p63 and p73, the p53 homologs, as tumor suppressors [Kaghad, 1997] and the fact that p73 is located in chromosome 1p36.3 frequently lost in NB tumors have attracted the attention of scientists who are anticipating the function of this gene in cancerogenesis. Hence, three proteins have been uncovered so far in the p53 superfamily of transcription factors: p53, p63, and p73. The two p53 homologs are similar to p53 in terms of structure and function but they are not identical owing to the complex structure of the gene (Figure 2). For example, p73 and p53 share the three functional domains: the transactivation (TA) domain, the DNA-binding domain (DBD) and the oligomerization domain (OD). A particular structural feature of the p73 gene is that full-length p73 (TAp73α) contains a sterile alpha motif (SAM) at the COOH-terminus. This has not been found in p53, but it has been found in other proteins known to be involved in the regulation of development [Levrero et al., 2000]. Of particular interest is the fact that p63 is involved in epithelial tissue development whereas p73 is instrumental for neural and hematopoietic tissue development. In addition, alternative splicing in the COOH-terminal region gives rise to a myriad of isoforms that serve various biological functions [Levrero et al., 2000] [Satoh et al., 2004]. At the NH2-terminus, the p73 gene harbors two distinct promoters that regulate the expression of two different classes of variants. The TAp73 variant is initiated from the P1 promoter and shares certain biological functions with p53, including the potential to induce a number of p53-responsive genes involved in growth arrest and the ability to trigger apoptosis [Kaghad et al., 1997]; [Jost et al., 1997]. The ΔNp73 variant, which lacks the TA, is initiated from the P2 promoter and can act as a dominant-negative protein by inhibiting the transcriptional activity of both p53 and TAp73 [Yang et al., 2000b]; [Fillippovich et al., 2001]. In this regard, ΔNp73 plays an essential anti-apoptotic role during neuron development as it can inhibit sympathetic neuron apoptosis following NGF withdrawal and rescue CNS neurons from various apoptotic stimuli upstream of caspase-3 activation [Pozniak et al., 2000]; [Pozniak et al., 2002]. More recently, it has been shown that ΔNp73α accumulates in differentiating monocytes of C2C12 cells and is able to protect them from apoptosis since its abrogation by siRNA-ΔNp73 leads to spontaneous apoptosis [Belloni et al., 2006].

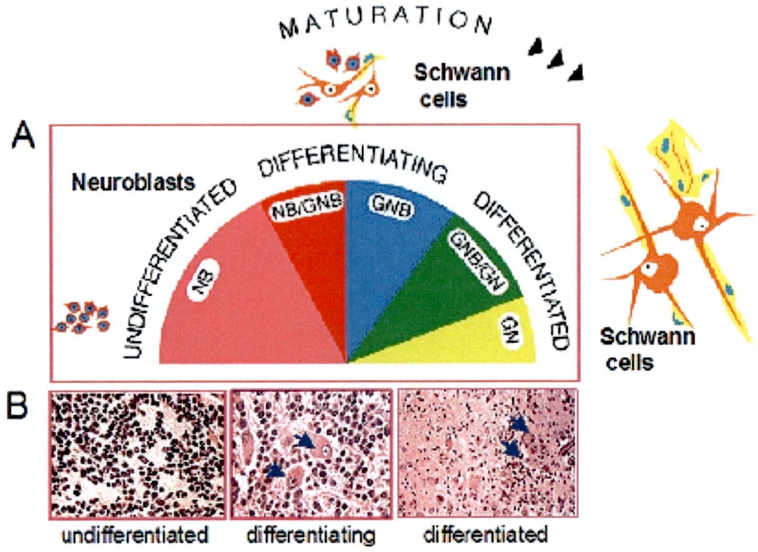

Figure 1. (A) Schematic representation of histological types of neuroblastic tumors according to the International Neuroblastoma Pathology Classification [Shimada et al., 1999] and classified according to their wide spectrum of differentiation. From left to right, the undifferentiated Schwannian stroma-poor subtype with immature NB cells to the well differentiated Schwannian stroma-dominant subtype labeled 'ganglioneuroma (GN) maturing subtype'. Between these two extremes lies a range of immature differentiating neuroblasts and mature ganglion cells comprising NB/GNB (ganglioneuroblastoma) and GNB/GN. (B) Hematoxylin-eosin staining of tissues from different NB patients showing different composites. Arrows indicate mature cells.

Our earlier work has demonstrated that the BTG2 promoter, known to be activated in neuronal differentiation, is specifically up-regulated by ΔNp73α in NB cells containing wtp53 but not in breast cancer MCF7 cells containing wtp53 [Goldschneider et al., 2005]. In other circumstances, TAp73α and p53 cooperate to induce strong apoptosis [Flores et al., 2002; Goldschneider et al., 2004; Goldschneider et al., 2003]. Additional complexity is arisen if we consider that TAp73 overexpression can induce ΔNp73α, which in turn regulates TAp73α/p53 through a feedback loop mechanism [Grob et al., 2001]; [Nakagawa et al., 2002].

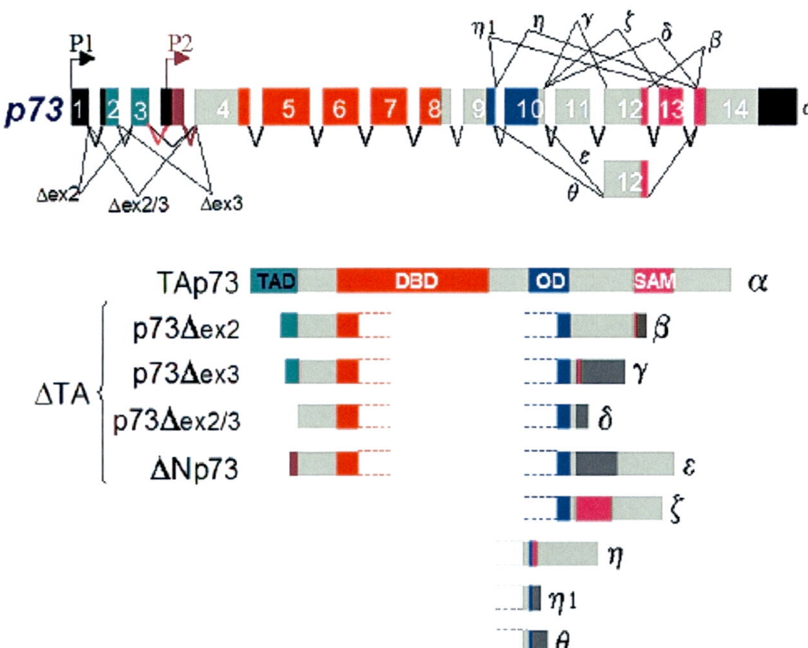

Figure 2. Structure and expression of the p73 gene. The p73 gene, like the p53 gene encodes protein which harbors three domains: the transactivation domain (TAD), the DNA binding domain (DBD), and the oligomerization domain (OD). In addition to these 3 domains, the p73 protein contains a sterile alpha motif (SAM) domain involved in protein-protein interactions in the C-terminal region. At the N-terminus, the p73 gene contains, in addition to the P1 promoter which regulates the translation of TAp73 isoforms, a second promoter, P2, located within intron 3 which encodes ΔNp73, an N-terminal truncated variant that lacks the TA domain. Other isoforms can be initiated from P1 but lack the TA domain to differing extents due to alternative splicings of exon 2 and/or 3. These isoforms are termed ΔTAp73. In addition to the alpha isoform, a variety of splice variants (β,χ, δ, ε, ζ,η,θ) resulting from alternative splicing have been reported at the C terminus.

In human NB tumors, we reported that the ΔNp73α isoform is the only p73 protein evidenced in poorly differentiated NB cells [Douc-Rasy et al., 2002]. This is consistent with the finding that ΔNp73 expression is associated with reduced apoptosis in NB tumor tissue and poor outcome [Casciano et al., 2002]. Several lines of evidence strongly point to p73 involvement in the development of the nervous system. Little, however, is known about their target genes in human NB tumors. The aim of our study was to investigate the gene expression profile of two human NB cell lines, SH-SY5Y containing endogenous wtp53 and IGR-N-91 containing mutated p53, both infected with either TAp73α or ΔNp73α recombinant adenoviruses. We used Clontech's Atlas Human Cancer 1.2 Array in our investigation.

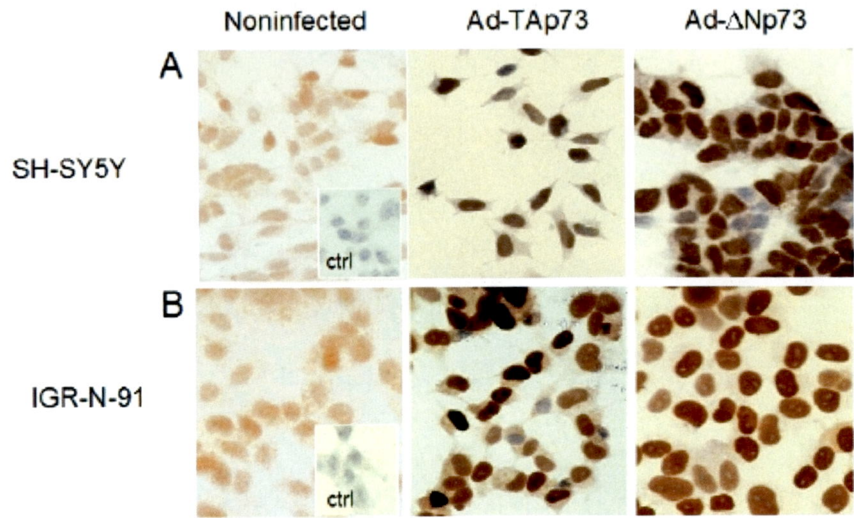

Figure 3. Immunocytochemistry study of SH-SY5Y (A) or IGR-N-91 (B) cells infected by recombinant adenovirus showing infection efficiency. The parental human NBSH-SY5Y cell line (ECACC, Wiltshire, UK) and IGR-N-91 (established in our laboratory) derived from multi-drug resistant patient were maintained in Dulbecco's Modified Eagle's Medium (DMEM). Forty-eight hours after infection, the cells were fixed in 4% paraformaldehyde. The fixed cells were hybridized with the rabbit polyclonal anti-p73α recognizing both TAp73α and ΔNp73α; proteins were revealed by ECL (Amersham) using the streptavidin-biotin method. The rabbit polyclonal p73 antibody raised against human p73 at the C-terminus (donated by Dr. D. Caput) was diluted at 1/280. A biotinylated anti-rabbit IgG and anti-mouse IgG (Dako) were used as secondary antibodies. Rabbit IgG and normal mouse IgG were used as negative controls in p73 experiments.

2. Identification and Classification of p73α-Target Genes

Gene Expression Profiles in Neuroblastoma Cell Lines by Macroarray Analysis

To define the potential interactivity between p73 and p53, we studied the gene expression profile in wt-p53 SH-SY5Y cells and compared it to that in mutated-p53 IGR-N-91 cells (duplication of p53 exons 7-8-9) [Goldschneider et al., 2004]. The SH-SY5Y and IGR-N-91 cells were infected with either TAp73α (Ad-TAp73α) or ΔNp73α (Ad-ΔNp73α) recombinant adenovirus at a multiplicity of infection of 15 viral particles per cell. Immunocytochemistry studies using p73 antibody showed an infection efficiency of nearly 100% in the nucleus of cells treated with recombinant adenovirus (Figures 3A and 3B). The cDNA macroarray experiments were conducted in duplicate using different filters. The Atlas Human Cancer filter 1.2 arrays (Clontech) contains 1176 different genes including oncogenes, tumor suppressor genes, cell cycle regulators, and transcription factors. When infected with TAp73, a number of genes were differentially up-regulated in SH-SY5Y cells when compared to IGRN-91 cells. Table 1 shows the results (ordered according to biological function) for the 14 TM bona fide target genes identified by cDNA macroarray analysis using AtlasImage2.0 software (Clontech). It can be seen that the most prominent target genes are associated with development and neuronal differentiation. MIC-1, a novel macrophage inhibitory cytokine 1, also known as GDF-15, is a divergent member of the transforming growth factor-beta superfamily that may act as an autocrine regulatory molecule as its expression is associated with cytokines such as TNF-α, which is secreted by activated macrophages [Bootcov et al., 1997]. MIC-1 has been found to be abundantly expressed by the choroid plexus [Strelau et al., 2000]. It may, therefore, play a key role in the central nervous system as both a neurotrophic and neuroprotective factor for midbrain dopaminergic neurons in vitro and in vivo. MIC-1 expression has been known to be regulated by environmental conditions in a spatiotemporal manner. For instance, MIC-1 prevents the death of cerebellar granule neurons (CGN) cultured in low K+. CGN can survive in high K+ for 25 minutes but undergoes apoptosis when switched to low K+ for 5 minutes [Subramaniam et al., 2003]. The results of the present study showed that MIC-1 was up-regulated by TAp73α in wtp53 SH-SY5Y cells and mutated p53 IGR-N-91 cells (5.2 vs 16.9 respectively). Expression levels were approximately 3 times higher in the mutated-p53 cells than in the wt-p53 cells; in contrast, MIC-1 was down-regulated by ΔNp73α (<2) in both cell types. Inversely, Notch1 and Jagged2 were only expressed, though abundantly, in SH-SY5Y cells. JAG2 protein encoded by Jagged2 is a ligand of the Notch1 receptor; the Notch1-JAG2 signaling pathways may function in vivo to coordinate the differentiation of certain groups of progenitor cells, and they may also modulate neuritic architecture [Luo et al., 1997]; [Franklin et al., 1999]. Members of the Notch family play a critical role as mediators in cell fate determination and maintenance of progenitors in many developmental systems [Milner et al., 1999]. A recent report by the Rulang Jiang group showed that in mice, Jagged2 played a critical role in oral epithelium tissue development and that Jagged2-Notch1 was spatiotemporally regulated to prevent unfavorable adhesion between oral tissues [Casey et al., 2006]. A number of up-regulated mRNAs encoding proteins involved in neural development are of particular interest. EphA2, a receptor tyrosine kinase, directs the differentiation of mammalian neural precursor cells, specifically in facilitating the neuritic extension of NB cells [Aoki et al., 2004], [Tanaka et al., 2004]. Wnt8A is known to be temporarily required by the Wnt signaling pathway during neural crest development. $p75^{NTR}$, a low-affinity nerve growth factor (NGF) receptor gene involved in neuronal development, and TrkA, a high-affinity tyrosine kinase receptor, are both cell surface receptors. Like TrkA, $p75^{NTR}$ can induce apoptosis following NGF withdrawal in neonatal culture sympathetic neurons [Aloyz et al., 1998]; [Nakagawara, 2001]. Although both TrkA and $p75^{NTR}$ have been recognized as p53 effectors that mediate apoptosis in response to NGF withdrawal, the role of $p75^{NTR}$ in neuronal differentiation remains unclear. In contrast, it is known to modulate TrkA affinity for NGF [Hempstead, 2002]. $p75^{NTR}$ mRNA levels have been found to be increased in CHP100 cells treated with basic fibroblast growth factor that induces morphologic changes and neurite outgrowth [Taiji et al., 1992]. More recently, [Zhang et al., 2005] demonstrated that $p75^{NTR}$ and TrkA expression were negatively correlated in human primary pancreatic cancers: while elevated $p75^{NTR}$ expression was associated with favorable prognosis, high expression levels of TrkA were a marker of unfavorable prognosis in pancreatic tumor patients but not in breast cancer patients.

In NB tumors, like in breast cancer, high levels of TrkA are associated with favorable prognosis [Eggert et al., 2002]. This contradictory function could be due to a short isoform (s-p75) that has been identified in mammals and birds. Animals lacking both isoforms exhibit a profound loss of sensory neurons and Schwann cells; they also exhibit more serious defects in terms of large blood vessel development and lack the full-length $p75^{NTR}$. This observation is consistent with the many faces of $p75^{NTR}$ reported so far [Hempstead, 2002]. The present study showed that $p75^{NTR}$ was more strongly up-regulated in wtp53 SH-SY5Y cells than in mutated p53 IGR-N-91 cells (5-fold increase), suggesting that $p75^{NTR}$ differential expression is p53 dependent. The Wnt8A gene involved in development was strongly up-regulated by both TAp73 and ΔNp73 in wt-p53 SH-SY5Y cells, suggesting that p53 may play a role as a mediator in this process. In a previous study, we saw that ΔNp73 specifically activated the BTG2 gene in NB

Table 1. Ratio of mRNA levels of p73-target genes in infected cells versus noninfected cells

Gene symbol	SH-SY5Ya		IGR-N-91b		Biological Function
	TAp73α	ΔNp73α	TAp73α	ΔNp73α	
MIC-1/GDF-15	5,2	<2	16,9	<2	
Notch1	9,2	<2	2	<2	
Jagged2	44,8	<2	2,3	<2	Development /
$p75^{NTR}$ (or $p75^{NGFR}$)	32,1	<2	6,1	<2	Neuronal Differentiation
IGFBP2	2,1	<2	2	<2	
EphrinA receptor 2	9,4	<2	2,9	<2	
Wnt8A	5,8	5,1	<2	<2	
Chromogranin B	2,1	<2	2,1	<2	Secretory granule Marker
PLGF	5,8	<2	<2	<2	Placental Growth Factor
Integrin α[illegible]3	8,9	<2	<2	<2	Cellular Adhesion
EGR1	2,9	<2	<2	<2	p53-Associated Transcription Factor
Cathepsin D	2,7	<2	2	<2	Lysosomal protease
p21WAF1	2,8	<2	15,7	<2	Cell Cycle Regulator
MDM2	<2	<2	2,2	<2	p53/TAp73 Regulator

Total RNA extracts were obtained from SH-SY5Y (wtp53) and IGR-N-91 (mutatedp53) cells infected with adenovirus expressing TAp73α or ΔNp73α. The labeling and hybridization procedures were conducted as specified by the manufacturer. cDNA probes were synthesized from 2.5 μg of total with [α-32P] dATP by oligo dT-primed polymerization using Superscript II reverse TM Transcriptase (Superscript II RNase H-, Gibco BRL Kit). Data derived from macroarray analyses were obtained from the mean value of two independent experiments. Only genes that showed at least a 2-fold up-(>2) or down-(>2) expression compared to the control were included in the analysis.

cells containing wtp53 [Goldschneider et al., 2005]. Yet, PC3 (the rat homolog of human BTG2) mRNA expression coincides both spatially and temporally with the pattern of CNS neurogenesis in the developing rat [Iacopetti et al., 1994].

Inhuman cells, BTG2 is known to be involved in cell growth, differentiation, and DNA repair, as well as the promotion of neuronal differentiation and the prevention of apoptosis of terminally differentiated cells [Tirone, 2001]; [el Ghissassi et al., 2002]. In addition to inducing developmental genes, TAp73α also induces a number of genes with diverse functions, the most noticeable being Integrin α3, which is more highly expressed in SH-SY5Y than in IGR-N-91 cells. This was validated by our RT-PCR analysis. It was reported very recently that, in certain circumstances, NB cells can promote survival during invasion when they lack caspase 8 yet retain integrin expression. In other circumstances, NB cells lacking caspase 8 and/or with decreased expression of integrin can promote metastasis [Stupack et al., 2006]. In addition, an in vitro study using TAp73-adenoviral infection showed that IGR-N-91 cells resisted apoptosis, whereas in a parallel experiment, all the SH-SY5Y cells died massively [Goldschneider et al., 2004]. The low expression levels of integrin α3 in IGR-N-91 cells may, therefore, be linked to its cellular invasion and metastasis capabilities given that these cells were derived from a patient with progressive disease characterized by MYCN amplification of up to 350 copies and high expression levels of MDR1 [Blanc et al., 2003]. Of the 14 genes identified as being differentially expressed (up-regulated) by macroarray analysis (Table 2), 7 were associated with development and differentiation. The others had different cell biology functions.

Genes Up-Regulated by p73α in p53-Mutated IGR-N-91 Cells

The histogram in Figure 4 shows the expression levels of several genes involved in development and neuronal differentiation in IGR-N-91 cells, including BTG2, ZO-1 (Zonula Occludens-1), tyrosinase and chromogranin B. Conventional TAp73-target genes such as p21, a cell cycle regulator, MDM2, a negative regulator of p53/p73, and GADD45, a gene involved in DNA repair, were strongly induced by TAp73, which is consistent with previous findings for NB cells under stress conditions [Goldschneider et al., 2004]; [Million et al., 2006].

ZO-1 has been previously identified in membrane proteins involved in signal transduction, and can interact with alpha-actinin-4-associated plasma membrane proteins to exhibit regulatory activities at cell-cell and cell-extracellular matrix contacts [Chen et al., 2006]. Notably, chromogranin B, a secretory granule protein marker of neuroendocrine cells, [Kimura et al., 2000] is recognized as being involved in sympathetic differentiation. The retinoblastoma-binding protein 3 (RBQ-3), a nuclear protein capable of binding to underphosphorylated pRb, was up-regulated when both isoforms of the p73 protein were overexpressed, yet it was more highly up-regulated by the N-truncated p73 isoform. This confirms that ΔNp73 plays a role in cellular proliferation. In contrast to other responsive genes, and in the presence of high p21 expression levels, the pro-apoptotic Bax gene was down-regulated. This is consistent with our previous FACS analysis, which demonstrated that TAp73α overexpression in mutated p53 IGR-N-91 cells induced cell cycle arrest but not apoptosis, and that TAp73α and p53 cooperated very efficiently in wt-p53 SH-SY5Y cells to trigger apoptosis [Goldschneider et al., 2004]. It is important to note that ΔNp73α represses a number of genes, in particular the S100 calcium-binding protein, S100A2, whereas expression is up-regulated during keratinocyte differentiation and down-regulated in response to TAp73α silencing [Lapi et al., 2006].

Table 2. Primer pairs used for RT-PCR

		Primer sequences (5' to 3')		
Gene No.	Accession	Forward	Reverse	PCR product size
*p75^NTR^*	M14764	ccgaggcaccaccgac	ggatgtggcagtggactcac	544 bp
MIC-1	AB000584	cggatactcacgccagaagtg	cccgagtccccaagaaggt	841 bp
Notch1	AF308602	tgcaggcaatccgaggacta	ggcaggcagtcgcagaa	278 bp
Jagged2	AF003521	cgatggctgcgggtca	tgtggcagggatcgggaag	296 bp
WNT8A	AB057725	catgtggtgagcaagtattact g	gctgctcttcagaagagactt	508 bp
Integrin α3	M59911	aggatgactgtgagcggatg	gcccgtctccaggtagtctg	287 bp
EphA2	M59371	tggctcacacacccgtatgg	gtggcgtgcctcgaagtc	354 bp
PGLF	X54936	ggtgcggcgatgctg	ggcccaagaacaggtagcag	379 bp

3. Analysis of Genes Induced by Adenoviral TAp73αor ΔNp73α Expression in NB Cells

To confirm the results of the macroarray analysis, we performed semi-quantitative RT-PCR analyses with an aliquot of RNA from 8 of the activated genes used for the macroarray analysis. As shown in Figure 5A, the transcript levels of the genes p75^{NTR}, MIC-1, Notch1, Jagged2, Wnt8A, Integrin α3, EphA2 and PGLF were consistent throughout with the expression profiles shown in Table 1. Of particular interest is the fact that RT-PCR confirmed that Wnt8A was strongly induced by TAp73α− and ΔNp73α−forced expression. As p73 is highly expressed in adrenal chromaffin cells – previously observed in an immunohistochemistry study of a tumor patient [Douc-Rasy et al., 2002] – and as chromogranin B is known to take part in intra-cellular homeostasis and to be abundantly expressed in adrenal chromaffin cells [Yoo et al., 2002; Lugardon et al., 2001], we subjected protein extracts from p73-adenovirus-infected NB cells to Western blot analysis. As can be seen in Figure 5B, chromogranin B was more highly induced by TAp73α in IGR-N-91 cells than in SH-SY5Y cells. As far as $p75^{NTR}$ induction is concerned, while the macroarray and RT-PCR data consistently corroborate each other, the luciferase data are far from clear. Indeed, in the SH-SY5Y cells, ΔNp73 α-and TAp73α−forced expression induced promoter activation in $p75^{NTR}$ but no transcript was revealed by ΔNp73α (Figure 5C vs Figure 5A and Table 1).

It is clear from the list in Table 1 and from Figures 4 and 5 that there is cross-talk between p53 and p73. Indeed, p73-responsive genes are differentially expressed according to cellular context. MIC-1 was highly induced in inactive-p53 IGR-N-91 cells, while other genes such as $p75^{NTR}$ and Notch1 were highly induced in wt-p53 cells. This supports the hypothesis that a concerted interaction may exist between p53 and p73.

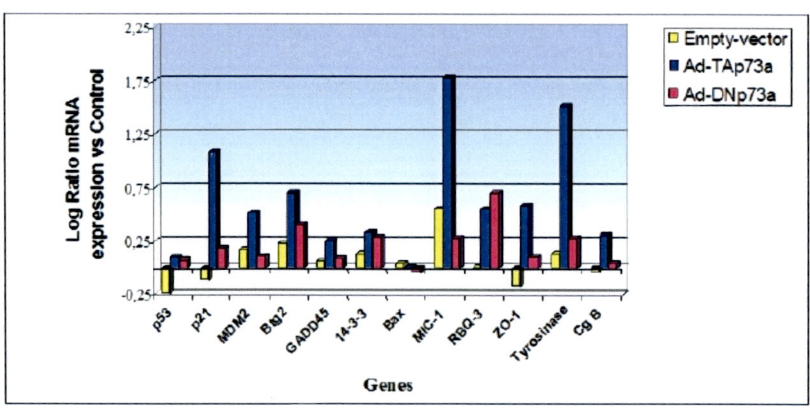

Figure 4. Histogram of expression levels of up-and down-regulated genes in IGR-N-91 infected cells compared to control cells. Logarithm of mRNA expression levels ratio of several p73-target genes in IGR-N-91 (inactive p53) cells transfected with either Ad-TAp73α (blue) or Ad-ΔNp73α (red).

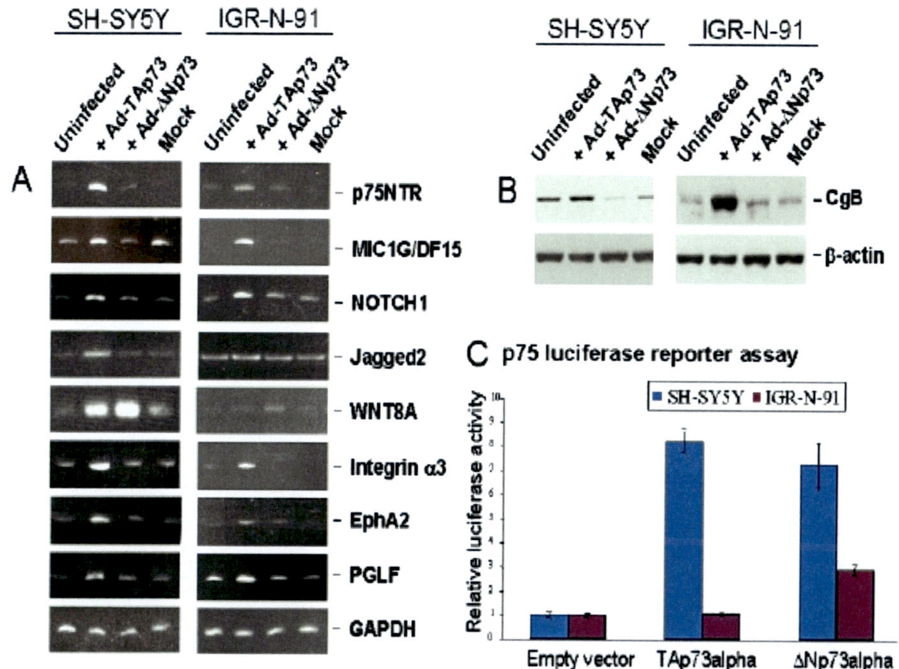

Figure 5. (A) Expression levels analysis of 8 induced genes by semi-quantitative RT-PCR using primer pairs in Table 2. To establish relative qualities, serial dilutions of cDNAs were amplified with GAPDH-specific primers (forward primer: 5'ctgcaccaccaactgcttag3'; reverse primer: 5'aggtccaccactgacacgtt for internal standardization). (B) Western blot analysis of chromogranin B (CgB) expression in SH-SY5Y and IGR-N-91 cells infected with TA-or ΔNp73. Antibody dilutions for immunoblotting were 1/50 for chromogranin B immunoblots (Astrocytes raised against chromogranin B were donated by Dr. Dominique Aunis, Strasbourg, France). (C) p75^{NTR} luciferase reporter assay. SH-SY5Y and IGR-N-91 cells were transfected with a reporter plasmid carrying 2.1kb promoter of p75^{NTR} (donated by Dr. Emil Bogenmann, Childrens Hospital, Los Angeles) with an expression vector (pcDNA-TAp73α or pcDNA-Δ Np73α plasmid). Twenty-four hours after transfection, the cells were lysed and luciferase activity was quantified as previously described (Goldschneider et al., 2005).

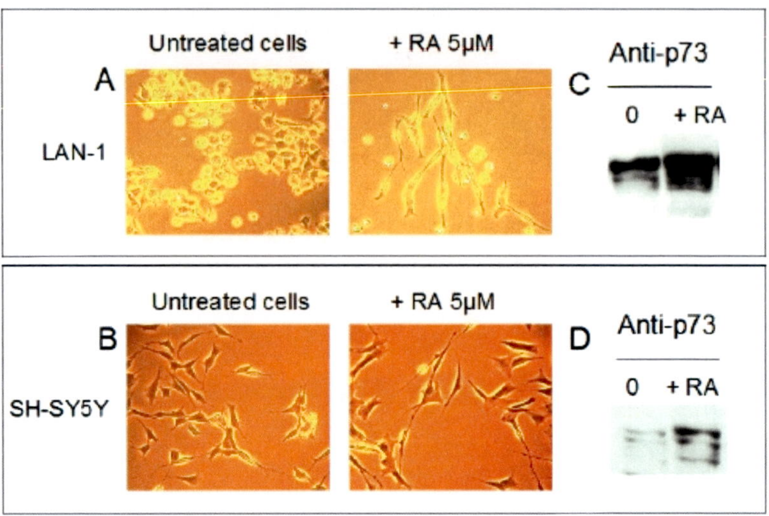

Figure 6. Morphology of LAN-1 (A) and SH-SY5Y (B) cells treated (or not) for 3 days with 5μM RA and Western blot (C) and (D) respectively. The LAN-1 cells were grown in RPMI medium.

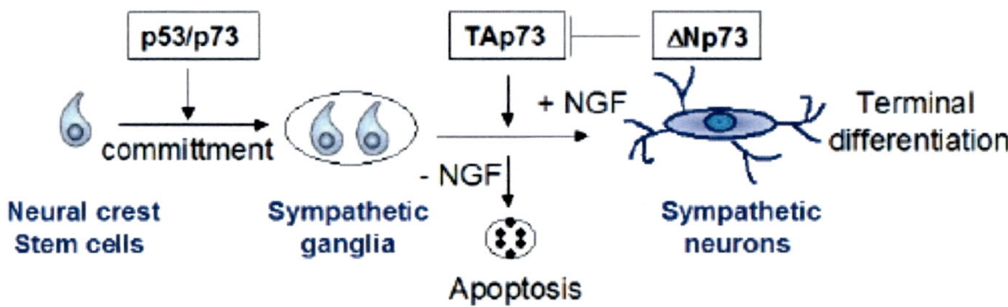

Figure 7. Scheme representing the possible involvement of p73 in neural development and differentiation of human malignant neuroblasts. In post-mitotic or cortical neurons, p53 is found to be increased following neural injury (Slack et al., 1996; Xiang et al., 1996). During nervous system development, the progenitor cells and post-mitotic neurons are overproduced. The p53 family plays an essential role in two key biological events, apoptosis and neuron survival, that are of prime necessity to ensure neuronal life and death (Miller et al., 2000). TAp73α is the predominant form in the developing brain where ΔNp73 elicits anti-apoptotic functions [Yang et al., 2000a]; [Pozniak et al., 2002]; [Meyer et al., 2004]. During development, the newly-born neurons migrate to their final destinations where TAp73α could be a principal mediator of apoptosis in 'unhealthy' neurons following NGF withdrawal. ΔNp73α, in contrast, operates with NGF to ensure the survival of 'healthy' neurons.

4. p73 Expression is Strongly Induced during Human NB Differentiation by Retinoic Acid

TAp73 involvement in NE115 mouse cell differentiation has been previously reported [De Laurenzi et al., 2000]. In order to explore the particular role of p73 in human NB cells, we treated LAN-1 cells expressing p73 but not p53 with all-trans retinoic acid (RA). As shown in Figure 6, all the malignant neuroblasts extended their neurites to establish appropriate connections, a process that is a recognized as functional marker of neuronal differentiation. The considerable accumulated production of TAp73α, shown by Western blot analysis, confirmed the implication of TAp73α in neuronal differentiation by RA (Figure 6A). Notably, p53 did not prevent neuritic extension, as the same morphology was observed in the SH-SY5Y cells expressing both p53 and p73 (Figure 6B). Conversely, the neuritic extension of NB cells by RA may not just depend on p53 or TAp73α transactivation as it also occurred in mutated-p53 IGR-N-91 cells without TAp73α.

5. Conclusion

The seminal work on p73 structure and function by the Caput group addresses the relationship between p73 and NB (Kaghad, 1997) given it revealed that p73 mapped on the 1p36.3 locus that is frequently deleted in NB tumors. The present study using adenovirus-mediated TAp73α and its variant ΔNp73α expression into NB cells revealed that half of the p73-target genes were associated with neuron development and differentiation. The study also showed that p53 and p73 either collaborated or interfered with one another according to the relevant development phases; more specifically, apoptosis and neuron survival, two key events physiologically required during neural development. As far as neuron development and differentiation are concerned, genes such as MIC-1/GDF-15 appear to be specifically induced by TAp73α, while others, such as Notch1 and Jagged 2 could be specifically triggered by p53. Collectively, our previous findings and those found in the literature point increasingly to the possibility that TAp73 plays a pivotal role in apoptosis in NB tumors. TAp73 cooperated efficiently with p53 for apoptosis in wt-p53 NB cells whereas it induced the up-regulation of genes involved in neuronal differentiation in the mutated-p53 cells. As a whole, p73 implication in stem cell identity, neurogenesis, natural immunity, and homeostatic control previously described in mice, is supported by the present human neuroblastoma study. In this regard, we identified p73 target-genes such as *Wnt8A* implicated in neural crest development, *MIC-1/GDF-15* in the central nervous system and Chromogranin B, due to its homeostasis control, in the physiological functioning of the sympathetic system. Nevertheless, the signaling pathways involving these genes have to be clearly demonstrated.

Reference List

Aloyz,R.S., Bamji,S.X., Pozniak,C.D., Toma,J.G., Atwal,J., Kaplan,D.R., and Miller,F.D. (1998). p53 is essential for developmental neuron death as regulated by the TrkA and p75 neurotrophin receptors. *J.Cell Biol.*, *143*, 1691-1703.

Aoki,M., Yamashita,T., and Tohyama,M. (2004). EphA receptors direct the differentiation of mammalian neural precursor cells through a mitogen-activated protein kinase-dependent pathway. *J. Biol. Chem.*, *279*, 32643-32650.

Belloni,L., D, Merlo,P., Damalas,A., Costanzo,A., Blandino,G., and Levrero,M. (2006). Np73alpha protects myogenic cells from apoptosis. *Oncogene*, *25*, 3606-3612.

Blanc,E., Goldschneider,D., Ferrandis,E., Barrois,M., Le Roux,G., Leonce,S., Douc-Rasy,S., Bénard,J., and Raguenez,G. (2003). MYCN enhances P-gp/MDR1 gene expression in the human metastatic neuroblastoma IGR-N-91 model. *Am. J. Pathol.*, *163*, 321-331.

Bootcov,M.R., Bauskin,A.R., Valenzuela,S.M., Moore,A.G., Bansal,M., He,X.Y., Zhang,H.P., Donnellan,M., Mahler,S., Pryor,K., Walsh,B.J., Nicholson,R.C., Fairlie,W.D., Por,S.B., Robbins,J.M., and Breit,S.N. (1997). MIC-1, a novel macrophage inhibitory cytokine, is a divergent member of the TGF-beta superfamily. *Proc. Natl. Acad. Sci.USA*, *94*, 11514-11519.

Casciano,I., Mazzocco,K., Boni,L., Pagnan,G., Banelli,B., Allemanni,G., Ponzoni,M., Tonini,G.P., and Romani,M. (2002). Expression of DeltaNp73 is a molecular marker for adverse outcome in neuroblastoma patients. *Cell Death.Differ.*, *9*, 246-251.

Casey,L.M., Lan,Y., Cho,E.S., Maltby,K.M., Gridley,T., and Jiang,R. (2006). Jag2-Notch1 signaling regulates oral epithelial differentiation and palate development. *Dev. Dyn.*, *235*, 1830-1844.

Chen,V.C., Li,X., Perreault,H., and Nagy,J.I. (2006). Interaction of Zonula Occludens-1 (ZO-1) with alpha-Actinin-4: Application of Functional Proteomics for Identification of PDZ Domain-Associated Proteins. *J. Proteome. Res.*, *5*, 2123-2134.

De Laurenzi, V., Raschella,G., Barcaroli,D., Annicchiarico-Petruzzelli,M., Ranalli,M., Catani,M.V., Tanno,B., Costanzo,A., Levrero,M., and Melino,G. (2000). Induction of neuronal differentiation by p73 in a neuroblastoma cell line. *J. Biol. Chem.*, *275*, 15226-15231.

Douc-Rasy,S., Barrois,M., Echeynne,M., Kaghad,M., Blanc,E., Raguenez,G., Goldschneider,D., Terrier-Lacombe,M.J., Hartmann,O., Moll,U., Caput,D., and Bénard,J. (2002). DeltaNp73alpha accumulates in human neuroblastic tumors. *Am. J. Pathol.*, *160*, 631-639.

Eggert,A., Grotzer,M.A., Ikegaki,N., Liu,X.G., Evans,A.E., and Brodeur,G.M. (2002). Expression of the neurotrophin receptor TrkA down-regulates expression and function of angiogenic stimulators in SH-SY5Y neuroblastoma cells. *Cancer Res.*, *62*, 18021808.

el Ghissassi,F., Valsesia-Wittmann,S., Falette,N., Duriez,C., Walden,P.D., and Puisieux,A. (2002). BTG2(TIS21/PC3) induces neuronal differentiation and prevents apoptosis of terminally differentiated PC12 cells. *Oncogene*, *21*, 6772-6778.

Fillippovich,I., Sorokina,N., Gatei,M., Haupt,Y., Hobson,K., Moallem,E., Spring,K., Mould,M., McGuckin,M.A., Lavin,M.F., and Khanna,K.K. (2001). Transactivationdeficient p73alpha (p73Deltaexon2) inhibits apoptosis and competes with p53. *Oncogene*, *20*, 514-522.

Flores,E.R., Tsai,K.Y., Crowley,D., Sengupta,S., Yang,A., McKeon,F., and Jacks,T. (2002). p63 and p73 are required for p53-dependent apoptosis in response to DNA damage. *Nature*, *416*, 560-564.

Franklin,J.L., Berechid,B.E., Cutting,F.B., Presente,A., Chambers,C.B., Foltz,D.R., Ferreira,A., and Nye,J.S. (1999). Autonomous and non-autonomous regulation of mammalian neurite development by Notch1 and Delta1. *Curr. Biol.*, *9*, 1448-1457.

Goldschneider,D., Blanc,E., Raguenez,G., Barrois,M., Legrand,A., Le Roux,G., Haddada,H., Bénard,J., and Douc-Rasy,S. (2004). Differential response of p53 target genes to p73 overexpression in SH-SY5Y neuroblastoma cell line. *J. Cell Sci.*, *117*, 293-301.

Goldschneider,D., Blanc,E., Raguenez,G., Haddada,H., Bénard,J., and Douc-Rasy,S. (2003). When p53 needs p73 to be functional - forced p73 expression induces nuclear accumulation of endogenous p53 protein.*Cancer Lett.*, *197*, 99-103.

Goldschneider,D., Million,K., Meiller,A., Haddada,H., Puisieux,A., Bénard,J., May,E., and Douc-Rasy,S. (2005). The neurogene BTG2TIS21/PC3 is transactivated by DeltaNp73alpha via p53 specifically in neuroblastoma cells. *J. Cell Sci.*, *118*, 12451253.

Grob,T.J., Novak,U., Maisse,C., Barcaroli,D., Luthi,A.U., Pirnia,F., Hugli,B., Graber,H.U., De,L., V, Fey,M.F., Melino,G., and Tobler,A. (2001). Human delta Np73 regulates a dominant negative feedback loop for TAp73 and p53. *Cell Death.Differ.*, *8*, 12131223.

Hempstead,B.L. (2002). The many faces of p75NTR. *Curr.Opin.Neurobiol.*, *12*, 260-267.

Iacopetti,P., Barsacchi,G., Tirone,F., Maffei,L., and Cremisi,F. (1994). Developmental expression of PC3 gene is correlated with neuronal cell birthday. *Mech. Dev.*, *47*, 127137.

Jost,C.A., Marin,M.C., and Kaelin,W.G., Jr. (1997). p73 is a simian [correction of human] p53related protein that can induce apoptosis. *Nature*, *389*, 191-194.

Kaghad,M., Bonnet,H., Yang,A., Creancier,L., Biscan,J.C., Valent,A., Minty,A., Chalon,P., Lelias,J.M., Dumont,X., Ferrara,P., McKeon,F., and Caput,D. (1997). Monoallelically expressed gene related to p53 at 1p36, a region frequently deleted in neuroblastoma and other human cancers. *Cell*, *90*, 809-819.

Kimura,N., Pilichowska,M., Okamoto,H., Kimura,I., and Aunis,D. (2000). Immunohistoche-mical expression of chromogranins A and B, prohormone convertases 2 and 3, and amidating enzyme in carcinoid tumors and pancreatic endocrine tumors. *Mod. Pathol.*, *13*, 140-146.

Lapi,E., Iovino,A., Fontemaggi,G., Soliera,A.R., Iacovelli,S., Sacchi,A., Rechavi,G., Givol,D., Blandino,G., and Strano,S. (2006). S100A2 gene is a direct transcriptional target of p53 homologues during keratinocyte differentiation. *Oncogene*, *25*, 36283637.

Levrero,M., De,L., V, Costanzo,A., Gong,J., Wang,J.Y., and Melino,G. (2000). The p53/p63/p73 family of transcription factors: overlapping and distinct functions. *J. Cell Sci.*, *113 (Pt 10)*, 1661-1670.

Lugardon,K., Chasserot-Golaz,S., Kieffer,A.E., Maget-Dana,R., Nullans,G., Kieffer,B., Aunis,D., and Metz-Boutigue,M.H. (2001). Structural and biological characterization of chromofungin, the antifungal chromogranin A-(47-66)-derived peptide. *J. Biol. Chem.*, *276*, 35875-35882.

Luo,B., Aster,J.C., Hasserjian,R.P., Kuo,F., and Sklar,J. (1997). Isolation and functional analysis of a cDNA for human Jagged2, a gene encoding a ligand for the Notch1 receptor. *Mol. Cell Biol.*, *17*, 6057-6067.

Meyer,G., Cabrera,S.A., Perez Garcia,C.G., Martinez,M.L., Walker,N., and Caput,D. (2004). Developmental roles of p73 in Cajal-Retzius cells and cortical patterning. *J. Neurosci.*, *24*, 9878-9887.

Million,K., Horvilleur,E., Goldschneider,D., Agina,M., Raguenez,G., Tournier,F., Bénard,J., and Douc-Rasy,S. (2006). Differential regulation of p73 variants in response to cisplatin treatment in SH-SY5Y neuroblastoma cells. *Int. J. Oncol.*, *29*, 147-154.

Milner,L.A. and Bigas,A. (1999). Notch as a mediator of cell fate determination in hematopoiesis: evidence and speculation. *Blood*, *93*, 2431-2448.

Moll,U.M.; Laquaglia,M.; Bénard,J.; Riou,G. (1995). Wild-type p53 protein undergoes cytoplasmic sequestration in undifferentiated neuroblastomas but not in differentiated tumors (1995). *Proc. Natl. Acad.. Sci 92*, 4407-4411.

Nakagawa,T., Takahashi,M., Ozaki,T., Watanabe,K.K., Todo,S., Mizuguchi,H., Hayakawa,T., and Nakagawara,A. (2002). Autoinhibitory regulation of p73 by Delta Np73 to modulate cell survival and death through a p73-specific target element within the Delta Np73 promoter. *Mol. Cell Biol.*, *22*, 2575-2585.

Nakagawara,A. (2001). Trk receptor tyrosine kinases: a bridge between cancer and neural development. *Cancer Lett.*, *169*, 107-114.

Nikolaev,A.Y., Li,M., Puskas,N., Qin,J., Gu,W. (2003). Parc: a cytoplasmic anchor for p53. *Cell, 112*, 29-40.

Ostermeyer,A.G. Runko,E., Winkfield,B., Ahn,B., Moll,U.M. (1996). Cytoplasmically sequestered wild-type p53 protein in neuroblastoma is relocated to the nucleus by a C-terminal peptide. *Proc. Natl. Acad. Sci. 93,* 15190-15194.

Pozniak,C.D., Barnabe-Heider,F., Rymar,V.V., Lee,A.F., Sadikot,A.F., and Miller,F.D. (2002). p73 is required for survival and maintenance of CNS neurons. *J. Neurosci.*, *22*, 98009809.

Pozniak,C.D., Radinovic,S., Yang,A., McKeon,F., Kaplan,D.R., and Miller,F.D. (2000). An anti-apoptotic role for the p53 family member, p73, during developmental neuron death. *Science*, *289*, 304-306.

Satoh,S., Arai,K., and Watanabe,S. (2004). Identification of a novel splicing form of zebrafish p73 having a strong transcriptional activity. *Biochem. Biophys. Res. Commun., 325*, 835-842.

Shimada,H., Ambros,I.M., Dehner,L.P., Hata,J., Joshi,V.V., and Roald,B. (1999). Terminology and morphologic criteria of neuroblastic tumors: recommendations by the International Neuroblastoma Pathology Committee. *Cancer, 86*, 349-363.

Strelau,J., Sullivan,A., Bottner,M., Lingor,P., Falkenstein,E., Suter-Crazzolara,C., Galter,D., Jaszai,J., Krieglstein,K., and Unsicker,K. (2000). Growth/differentiation factor15/macrophage inhibitory cytokine-1 is a novel trophic factor for midbrain dopaminergic neurons in vivo. *J. Neurosci., 20*, 8597-8603.

Stupack,D.G., Teitz,T., Potter,M.D., Mikolon,D., Houghton,P.J., Kidd,V.J., Lahti,J.M., and Cheresh,D.A. (2006). Potentiation of neuroblastoma metastasis by loss of caspase-8. *Nature, 439*, 95-99.

Subramaniam,S., Strelau,J., and Unsicker,K. (2003). Growth differentiation factor-15 prevents low potassium-induced cell death of cerebellar granule neurons by differential regulation of Akt and ERK pathways. *J. Biol. Chem., 278*, 8904-8912.

Taiji,M., Taiji,K., Deyerle,K.L., and Bothwell,M. (1992). Basic fibroblast growth factor enhances nerve growth factor receptor gene promoter activity in human neuroblastoma cell line CHP100. *Mol. Cell Biol., 12*, 2193-2202.

Tanaka,M., Ohashi,R., Nakamura,R., Shinmura,K., Kamo,T., Sakai,R., and Sugimura,H. (2004). Tiam1 mediates neurite outgrowth induced by ephrin-B1 and EphA2. *EMBO J., 23*, 1075-1088.

Tirone,F. (2001). The gene PC3(TIS21/BTG2), prototype member of the PC3/BTG/TOB family: regulator in control of cell growth, differentiation, and DNA repair? *J. Cell Physiol, 187*, 155-165.

Yang,A., Walker,N., Bronson,R., Kaghad,M., Oosterwegel,M., Bonnin,J., Vagner,C., Bonnet,H., Dikkes,P., Sharpe,A., McKeon,F., and Caput,D. (2000a). p73-deficient mice have neurological, pheromonal and inflammatory defects but lack spontaneous tumours. *Nature, 404*, 99-103.

Yang,H.W., Piao,H.Y., Chen,Y.Z., Takita,J., Kobayashi,M., Taniwaki,M., Hashizume,K., Hanada,R., Yamamoto,K., Taki,T., Bessho,F., Yanagisawa,M., and Hayashi,Y. (2000b). The p73 gene is less involved in the development but involved in the progression of neuroblastoma. *Int. J. Mol. Med., 5*, 379-384.

Yoo,S.H., You,S.H., Kang,M.K., Huh,Y.H., Lee,C.S., and Shim,C.S. (2002). Localization of the secretory granule marker protein chromogranin B in the nucleus. Potential role in transcription control. *J. Biol. Chem., 277*, 16011-16021.

Zhang,Y., Dang,C., Ma,Q., and Shimahara,Y. (2005). Expression of nerve growth factor receptors and their prognostic value in human pancreatic cancer. *Oncol.Rep., 14*, 161171.

The first two authors contributed equally to this work

In: Neuroblastoma Research Trends
Editors: L. H. Andre and N. E. Roux
ISBN: 978-1-60456-790-8

Chapter V

The Relationships are between the Neuroblastome and Caspases 3, 8, 9

***Jianghua Zhan*[*,1], *Liqin Zhang*[2] *and Hong Lin*[3]**
1. General Pediatric Surgery, Associate Professor, Tianjin Medical University, Tianjin Children's Hospital
2. Department of Gynecologic cytology, Tianjin General Hospital, Tianjin Medical University
3. Department of Pediatric Surgery, Tianjin Children's Hospital

Neuroblastoma (NB), one of the common malignant childhood tumors, arises from neuroblast cells derived from the neural crest and destined for the adrenal medulla and the sympathetic nervous system and affects approximately 1 in 100,000 individuals. NB represents 7% to 10% of all malignancies diagnosed in pediatric patients younger than 15 years of age and is responsible for approximately 15% of all pediatric cancer deaths [1]. However, NB is a heterogeneous disease; tumors can spontaneously regress or mature, or display a very aggressive, malignant phenotype. Because of these unique characteristics, NB has been of great interest to both clinicians and basic scientists. Progress in

[*] Contact Address: Jianghua Zhan, MD, Ph.D. Department of Pediatric Surgery, Tianjin Children's Hospital, Tianjin, P. R. China, 300074.

molecular and cellular biology and immunology in the past 10 years has contributed greatly to a better understanding of this disease; however, this progress has not significantly altered the clinical outcome for patients with NB. Cell apoptotic has been characterized by a progressive series of morphological and biochemical changes, it is a mechanism that organisms utilize to eliminate no need cells. Research shows the programmed cell death or apoptosis and its controlling gene abnormality is one of the main causes of tumor mechanism. Caspases protease families are Cysteinyl Aspartate Specific Protease（Caspase） plays a very important role in cancer apoptosis.

Chromosomal structural changes play a role in NB, particularly those that result in the loss of tumor suppressors, or gain of oncogenes, gene amplication, and activating or inactivating mutations of relevant genes or their regulatory elements [2]. The end result of alterations in these genetic elements, regardless of their specific mechanisms, is the disruption of the normal balance between cell proliferation and cell death. It has been known for many years that NBs show remarkable biologic heterogeneity, resulting in favorable prognosis in some instances and unfavorable prognosis owing to aggressive growth despite multimodal. Also noted on early karyotype analyses of NB derived cell lines were frequent deletions of the short arm of chromosome 1. deletions of genetic material in tumors suggest the presence of a tumor suppressor gene has been identified on chromosome 1p. functional confirmation of the presence of a 1p tumor suppressor gene came from the demonstration that transfection of chromosome 1p into a NB cell line results in morphologic changes and ultimately cell senescence [3]. That is the caspase-9 chromosome location [4].

Caspases cleave numerous substrates at the carboxyl side of an aspirate residue upon induction of apoptosis. A key caspase involved in the apoptotic pathway is caspase-3 (also known as Yama, CPP32, and Apopain). Our experience also testified that the expression of Caspase-3 in NB was higher than that of paraganglioma (GN) and normal adrenal tissue ($P<0.05$). Inhibition of caspase-3 has been linked to prevention of apoptotic death in vitro [5], although certain stimuli can induce apoptosis by a caspase-3 independent pathway. From a mechanistic point of view, while caspase-3 deficiencies probably causes an impairment of the entire apoptotic process, the cancer advantage related to caspase-8 absences is less straightforward [6]. It has been demonstrated a few years ago, however, that caspase-8, not caspase-3, is involved in the transcription-independent death process activated by p53 protein [7]. Thus, the absence of caspase-8 might confer two distinct advantages to NB cells: 1) it decreases the anti-tumoral immunological response because of the engagement of cell death receptors (by Fas ligand, tumor necrosis factor, and TRAIL), and 2) it down-regulates p53- mediated transcription-independent apoptosis, it is also intriguing that NBs express a high level of survivin gene [8].

Survivin is an anti-apoptotic protein that inhibits caspase-3 and 7 activation and thus protects neoplasias against anticancer treatment on the basis of cell death mechanisms. Considering the data on caspases-3 and 8 and those reported on survivin gene expression [8], it seems probable that NBs have developed a large variety of anti-apoptotic strategies that may be responsible for the resistance of this cancer to treatment. Recent observations have demonstrated that survivin inhibits apoptosis induced by a variety of agents by interfering with caspase-9 activation [9]. Cleavage of caspase-9 occurs during TRAIL-induced apoptosis, suggesting that survivin may contribute to the regulation of this event. Survivin acts as a mitotic substrate of the cyclin-dependent kinase p34cdc2-cyclin B1, and phosphorylation of survivin may regulate apoptosis at cell division by neutralizing caspase-9 [9]. Caspase-9 is part of an evolutionary conserved "apoptosome" complex that induces down-stream activation of effector caspase in the mitochondrial pathway of apoptosis. Dissociation of a survivin-caspase-9 complex on the mitotic apparatus led to caspase-9–dependent apoptosis of cells traversing mitosis [10]. These observations suggest that survivin plays an important role in cell proliferation and thus its expression in tumors of higher grade, and worse prognosis would compliment its proposed function as an anti-apoptotic protein at the interface between apoptosis and tumor cell division.

The caspase-*8* gene is located at chromosome locus 2q33, a region of loss of heterozygosity in several cancers including NB [11]. It was therefore possible that the absence of expression of caspase-8 observed in N-type cells and stage IV tumors was due to a homozygous deletion at this locus. Mutation of caspase-8 is an infrequent finding in cell lines or tumor samples; however, the loss of caspase-8 gene expression caused by hypermethylation of the caspase-8 promoter region has been found in a large percentage of NBs and that Non–caspase-8–expressing NB cells were found to be resistant to death-receptor–mediated apoptosis. In certain aggressive NBs, signal transduction, as exemplified by loss of caspase-8 expression, is found to be defective [12]. Our experience demonstrated that the expression of Caspase-8 in both of GN and normal adrenal tissue was higher than in that of Ganglio-Neuroblastoma (GNB) and NB ($P<0.01$), and there are different expression of caspase-8 in different clinical stages. Furthermore, the expression of Caspase-3,8 was related to clinical stage in NB, favorable histological categories (I+II+IVs) was higher than unfavorable histological categories (III+IV) ($P<0.05$).

Malignant NB cells lack caspase-8 expression, which correlates to their tumorigenicity and resistance to tumor-selective ligand tumor necrosis factor-related apoptosis-inducing ligand (TRAIL) and may be due to hypermethylation of the caspase-8 promoter [13]. In contrast, noninvasive NB cells express caspase-8 and are susceptible to TRAIL. Caspase-8 down-regulation may explain the aggressive behavior of high-stage NB, whereas the high sensitivity of noninvasive NB cells to TRAIL may account for the spontaneous regression of low-stage. Absence of caspase-8 in malignant NB cells tumors *in vivo*. Combined therapy including TRAIL and agents such as AzaC that induce in caspase-8 expression may be more successful, in addition to treatment with agents that induce apoptosis via caspase-8-independent mechanisms.

IFN- induces procaspase-8 expression in NB cells and that this induction is not dependent on demethylation of caspase-8 promoter sequence [14]. This finding is important because it suggests that re-expression of genes silenced by hypermethylation is not only dependent on demethylation but may also involve other mechanisms that may bypass hypermethylation. These data also suggest that therapies aimed at inducing caspase-8 expression by adjunctive IFN- treatment may increase the effectiveness of current chemotherapeutic regimen. Thus, caspase-8 acts as an initiator caspase that can activate the downstream effector caspases in the apoptotic cascade in response to the activation of death receptors, eventually resulting in apoptosis.

Elankumaran [15] identify the mechanistic events leading to apoptosis when tumor cells are infected with Newcastle disease virus (NDV). They have demonstrated that apoptosis is initiated by rNDV through the mitochondrial intrinsic pathway, leading to the activation of caspase-9 and effector caspase-3. A second round of caspase activation occurs when TRAIL-induced death receptor-mediated or caspase-3-mediated caspase-8 activation commences.

Caspase-8 amplifies the cycle, allowing full expression of apoptosis leading to oncolysis. While caspase-8 may play a role in amplifying effector's caspase activation, this appears to be unnecessary for NDV-induced apoptosis. The delay in TRAIL expression also supports this view. Reoviruses induce apoptosis primarily through the death receptor pathway, and cytochrome *c* release and subsequent caspase-9 activation were not critical mitochondrial events in apoptosis induction [16]. NDV, on the other hand, depends primarily on the mitochondrial apoptotic pathway with no dependence on the death receptor pathway, which suggests that the molecular mechanisms of apoptosis may depend on the virus strain and cell type.

At recently, Bozzo [17] demonstrated that SK-N-BE cells anoikis requires caspase-8 and -3 involvement, respectively as upstream and downstream caspases, without involving caspase-9. Although the biochemical activation pattern of this caspase has been seen functionally intact in SK-N-BE, as starvation experiments have evidenced. The absence of caspase-9 involvement in anoikis may be unexpected, since it was reported that caspase-9 could be activated by derangement of mitochondrion or by proteolytic action of caspase-8 itself.

In conclusion, the deficiency of caspase-3, 8 was found in unfavorable histological categories NB specimens. Moreover, the lack of caspase-8 may be correlated with negative prognostic features. Expression of Capase-9 in GN was higher than that of NB; casepase-9 gene is not subject to single somatic mutations and does not behave as a classical tumor suppressor gene in NB tumors. Epigenetic silencing of caspases has been proposed to regulate the tumor suppressor potential of caspases. Therapies aimed at inducing caspase-8 expression by adjunctive IFN- treatment may increase the effectiveness of current chemotherapeutic regimen. Future investigations will evaluate the importance of these current observations in NB development and in the planning of new therapy based on the forced re-expression of caspase genes.

Reference

[1] Young JL, Ries LG, Silverberg E, et al: Cancer incidence, survival, and mortality for children younger than 15 years. *Cancer*.1986; 58: 598-602.

[2] Oldham KT, Colombani PM, Foglia RP, et al: *Principles and Practice of Pediatric Surgery*. 2005, 571-594.

[3] Bader SA, Fasching C, Brodeur GM, et al: Dissociation of suppression of tumorigenicity and differentiation in vitro effected by transfer of single human chromosomes into human neuroblastoma cells. *Cell Growth Differ*. 1991; 2: 245-255.

[4] Shinji Hadano, Jamal Nasir, Kerrie Nichol: Genomic organization of the human caspase-9 gene on Chromosome 1p36.1-p36.3 *Mammalian Genome* 10, 757–760 (1999).

[5] Nicholson DW, Ali A, Thornberry NA, Vaillancourt JP, Ding CK, Gallant M, Gareau Y, Griffin PR, Labelle M, Lazebnik YA et al. Identification and

inhibition of the ICE/CED-3 protease necessary for mammalian apoptosis. *Nature* 1995; 376: 37–43.

[6] Achille Iolascona, Adriana Borriellob, Lucia Giordanic, Caspase 3 and 8 deficiency in human neuroblastoma. *Cancer Genetics and Cytogenetics.* 146 (2003) 41–47.

[7] Ding H-F, Lin Y-L, McGill G, Juo P, Zhu H, Blenis J, Yuan J, Fisher DE. Essential role for caspase-8 in transcription-independent apoptosis triggered by p53. *J. Biol. Chem.* 2000; 275:38905–11.

[8] Adida C, Berrebi D, Peuchmaur M, Reyes-Mugica M, Altieri DC. Anti-apoptosis gene, survivin, and prognosis of neuroblastoma. *Lancet* 1998;351:882–3.

[9] O'Connor DS, Grossman D, Plescia J, et al. Regulation of apoptosis at cell division by p34cdc2. *Proc. Natl. Acad. Sci. USA* 2000; 97:13103 - 7.

[10] Seol D-W, Billiar TR. A caspase-9 variant missing the catalytic site is an endogenous inhibitor of apoptosis. *J. Biol. Chem.* 1999, 274, 2072–2076.

[11] Hopkins-Donaldson S, Bodmer JL, Bourloud KB, et al: Loss of caspase-8 expression in highly malignant human neuroblastoma cells correlates with resistance to tumor necrosis factor-related apoptosis- inducing ligand-induced apoptosis. *Cancer Res.* 60: 4315-4319, 2000.

[12] Tal Teitz Jill M. Lahti Vincent J. Kidd Aggressive childhood neuroblastomas do not express caspase-8: an important component of programmed cell death *J. Mol. Med.* (2001) 79: 428–436.

[13] Teitz T, Wei T, Valentine MB, et al. Caspase 8 is deleted or silenced preferentially in childhood neuroblastomas with amplification of N-MYC. *Nature Med.* 2000, 6, 529–535.

[14] Kim, S, Kang J, Mark Evers B, et al: Interferon-Induces Caspase-8 in Neuroblastomas without Affecting Methylation of Caspase-8 Promoter. *J. Pediatr. Surg.* 2004, 39 (4), 509-515.

[15] Elankumaran S, Rockemann D, and Samal S: Newcastle Disease Virus Exerts Oncolysis by both Intrinsic and Extrinsic Caspase-Dependent Pathways of Cell Death. *J. Viro.,* Aug. 2006, p7522–7534.

[16] D.R. Catchpoole, R.B. Lock: The potential tumour suppressor role for caspase-9(CASP9) in the childhood malignancy, neuroblastoma. *European Journal of Cancer* 37 (2001) 2217–2221.

[17] C. Bozzo, Sabbatini M, Tiberio R et al. Activation of caspase-8 triggers anoikis in human neuroblastoma cells. *Neuroscience Research* 56 (2006) 145–153.

In: Neuroblastoma Research Trends
Editors: L. H. Andre and N. E. Roux
ISBN: 978-1-60456-790-8

Chapter VI

Genome and Proteome in Neuroblastoma

K. Gana[1], M. Moschovi, G. I. Lambrou and F. Tzortzatou-Stathopoulou[1,*]
1. Hematology/Oncology Unit University of Athens "Aghia Sophia" Children's Hospital, Goudi 11527 Athens HELLAS

Introduction Genome in Neuroblastoma [NB]

Pediatric neuro-ectodermal tumors range from undifferentiated, truly malignant neuroblastomas, via ganglioneuroblastomas to well-differentiated, mostly benign ganglioneuromas. Within the group of malignant neuroblastomas, different risk categories can be identified: patients with high, intermediate or low risk tumors. High-risk tumors include disseminated disease or bulky tumors with gross genetic alterations, such as the amplification of the oncogene MYCN [1] (INSS stages 3 and 4).

A number of biologic variables have been studied in children with neuroblastoma. Of particular importance are Shimada histology, aneuploidy of

[*] Prof. Fotini Tzortzatou-Stathopoulou, MD PhD Hematology/Oncology Unit University of Athens "Aghia Sofia" Childrens Hospital, Goudi 11527 Athens HELLAS ftzortza@med.uoa.gr.

tumor DNA, and amplification of the MYCN oncogene within tumor tissue, since treatment decisions may be based on these factors [2-8]. Gains and losses of one or more chromosomes of the diploid genome (aneuploidy) is a form of genetic instability frequently observed in neuroblastomas. Near-diploid and near-tetraploid tumors are usually detected in patients over 1 year of age. They are associated with structural abnormalities involving allelic loss of chromosome 1p, amplification of the MYCN gene and also, with aggressive tumors and dismal outcome. Hyperdiploid or near-triploid tumors are usually found in patients under the age of 12 months or in low-risk tumors (stages 1, 2 and 4s) with few or no structural chromosomal abnormalities i.e. hyperdiploid tumor DNA is associated with a favorable prognosis [9], especially in infants with neuroblastoma [5]. Near-pentaploid tumors are rare and found in patients with favorable prognostic factors and excellent prognosis, as in near-triploid tumors [10]. The mechanism(s) leading to this form of genetic instability in human cancers or neuroblastomas is still unclear. In general, incorrect segregation of chromatids and aneuploidy are considered to result from amplification or hypertrophia of centrosomes [11].

Amplification of the proto-oncogene MYCN is the most prototypic genetic aberration in neuroblastomas and is found in 20–25% of all neuroblastomas. MYCN was identified as a gene homologous to c-MYC and over represented in neuroblastomas. Amplified MYCN sequences usually form double minute (dmins) chromosomes or homogeneously staining regions (HSRs), which contain 50–500 copies of the MYCN gene.

MYCN gene amplification is associated with a poor prognosis regardless of patient age [4,5,12] Amplification of MYCN is associated with deletion of chromosome 1p and gain of the long arm of chromosome 17(17q), the latter of which independently predicts a poor prognosis [13, 14]. A higher proportion of proliferating tumor cells may independently predict poor prognosis [15]. In tumors with amplification of MYCN, LOH of 1p usually affects large areas, often reaching to 1p32 or even more proximal. The shortest region of overlap (SRO) for MYCN amplified tumors has been defined to 1p35–1pter [16]. This defect is strongly associated with dismal outcome. In contrast, the SRO for 1p deletions in MYCN single copy tumors was found to be smaller, and defined at 1p36.3 [17, 18]. The different regions of deletion associated with different biological entities suggest the existence of more than one tumor suppressor gene at chromosome 1p. Expression of the gene encoding one of the high-affinity neurotrophin receptors (termed TrkA, a nerve growth factor receptor), is associated with good prognosis tumors [19]. Increased levels of telomerase RNA [20], elevated serum ferritin [21], elevated serum lactate dehydrogenase [22], and the persistence of neuroblastoma cells in bone marrow during or after chemotherapy are each associated with poor prognosis [7, 21-28]. Biologic staging consisting of MYCN copy number and age is useful in defining prognosis and treatment of neuroblastoma [8, 29].

Neuroblastoma has been categorized into 3 biological groups. One type expresses the TrkA neurotrophin receptor, is hyperdiploid, and tends to spontaneously regress. Another type expresses the TrkB neurotrophin receptor; has gained an additional chromosome, 17q; has loss of heterozygosity of 14q; and is genomically unstable. In a third type, chromosome 1p is lost and the MYCN gene becomes amplified [30, 31]. MYCN amplification is currently used for the identification of high-risk patients and is implemented in all international clinical trials for the treatment stratification of neuroblastoma patients.

Spontaneous regression of neuroblastoma has been well described in infants, especially in those with the 4S pattern of metastatic spread [31, 32]. Regression generally occurs only in tumors with a near triploid number of chromosomes that also lack MYCN amplification and loss of chromosome 1p. Features associated with spontaneous regression include the lack of expression of telomerase [33, 34], expression of the ras family genes [35], and expression of the neurotrophin receptor TrkA. Recent studies have suggested that selected infants who appear to have asymptomatic, small, low-stage neuroblastoma detected by screening, often have tumors that spontaneously regress and may be observed safely without surgical intervention or tissue diagnosis [36].

From Genome to Proteome

In the past decade, new methods for quantitative high-throughput analysis of genes, transcripts and proteins have been introduced and applied in the field of cancer genetics. It has been demonstrated that genome wide detection of DNA low copy number changes is feasible using comparative genomic hybridization (CGH) arrays [37, 38]. At the mRNA level, gene expression profiling has become feasible through the introduction of cDNA [39] and oligonucleotide microarrays [40], which allow simultaneous analysis of thousands of genes. Real-time quantitative polymerase chain reaction (Q-PCR) has evolved the new standard for accurate quantification selected subsets of gene specific DNA or RNA sequences [41]. In parallel with the genomics and transcriptomics research areas, proteomics is also coming to the forefront of cancer research as a result of new and powerful analytical methods.

Scientists have already taken on the next great challenge to compile structural and functional data for all proteins expressed in an organism, tissue, body fluid or cell i.e. the proteome [42]. This challenge is currently addressed by the integrated efforts of genomics, proteomics, transcriptomics and metabolomics i.e. the study of the complement of genes, proteins, mRNA species and metabolites, present in a cell under defined conditions. A holistic understanding of protein function and structure will have an immense impact on disease diagnosis, drug development and our self-knowledge surpassing that of the genome era.

In contrast to MYCN gene amplification, the degree of expression of the MYCN gene in the tumor does not predict prognosis [43, 44], but it has been shown that the overexpression of transfected MYCN in cultured mammalian cells strongly increases proliferation rates and is able to induce cellular transformation [45, 46]. Studies carried out in transgenic mice with overexpression of MYCN gene in neural crest-derived tissues indicate the frequent development of neuroblastomas [47]. Also, the reduction of MYCN mRNA by the use of antisense MYCN can decrease proliferation and/or induce differentiation in cultured human neuroblastoma cell lines [48].

The MYCN product (MYCN) is a nuclear phosphoprotein, which can transcriptionally activate many genes, either directly (e.g. ID2) or indirectly [49].

A recent DNA microarray analysis suggested there is a link between DNA methylation and MYCN gene expression i.e. there is evidence DNA methylation may directly control MYCN oncoprotein levels [50]. Epigenetic silencing of potential tumor suppressor genes as an alternative mechanism in the absence of genetic mutations has not yet been studied systematically in neuroblastomas and needs further investigation.

Detection of *MYCN*

Neuroblastoma tumors show remarkable biological heterogeneity. Therefore to predict the biological behavior of an individual tumor and the prognosis of neuroblastoma patients, several parameters have been proposed. These include DNA ploidy and deletion of the short arm of chromosome 1, MYCN gene amplification and TrkA expression and telomerase activity [39].

In view of the importance of accurate assessment of these biological parameters, a recent quality control study of the SIOP Europe Neuroblastoma

Biology Group recommended the investigation of MYCN amplification and 1p-deletion using a second independent technique in parallel with fluorescence in situ hybridization (FISH).

The use of molecular analysis as a prognostic factor relies on the simplicity, reliability and the rapidity of the chosen procedure. The detection of gene amplification can be carried out using FISH [51] and Southern blotting (SB) techniques, both of which require a significant amount of high quality DNA and several days in order to obtain the results. Sometimes the samples obtained by aspiration or biopsy are small and other times archival paraffin embedded tissue may be used, making it difficult to obtain enough quantity/quality of DNA. In cases where the assay is required in order to determine the appropriate therapeutic regimen, the above techniques are unsuitable since they are not rapid.

The Polymerase Chain Reaction (PCR) and the Reverse Transcription PCR (RT-PCR) are powerful procedures for the amplification of small amounts of DNA or mRNA, respectively, for molecular analysis. These procedures are efficient since they require only small amounts of sample, are rapid and in the case of PCR even partially degraded DNA can be used. The downside of these techniques is the fact that in both cases the results are qualitative. Therefore the exact gene copy number of MYCN cannot be evaluated with the PCR technique.

Another advanced technique, based on the PCR, that can be used to produce quantitative results, is that of the Real Time PCR (Q-PCR). Q-PCR offers major advantages compared to conventional methods such as Southern blotting (SB) and former simple PCR. The advantages of real time PCR are the large dynamic range of quantification, the exclusion of post-PCR manipulations, the possibility to perform the assay on minimal amounts of tumor material (such as needle biopsies), the speed and the high throughput capacity (e.g. for retrospective studies on many samples) [44, 51, 52, 53].

We have developed a Q-PCR assay based on two different detection chemistries (i.e. SYBR Green I and Hyprobes) for the detection of amplified MYCN (unpublished data). SYBR Green is a fluorescent dye with which dNTP's are labeled in this system. Therefore the amplified DNA is labeled with the dye and the products of the reaction are detected and identified, at the end of each PCR cycle, by their melting point (Tm). In the second system, two oligonucleotide probes labeled with Fluorescein and LC Red, respectively, bind specifically to the product once formed.

Upon binding of the probes, there is a transfer of energy between them, detected as fluorescence. Therefore in this case the amplified DNA is monitored at the end of each PCR cycle by directly counting the fluorescence emitted by the annealed probes.

The housekeeping gene b-globin was used as a control for the reaction while normal genomic DNA and DNA extracted from the cell line Kelly (100-fold amplified MYCN) was used as the negative and positive controls for the reaction, respectively. Initially, qualitative PCR experiments were carried out to confirm the optimal parameters for the oligonucleotide primers (Figure 1). The results suggest that both methods can be used for the prognosis of neuroblastoma in patients since they ultimately confirm one another, are cost-effective, rapid and accurate (Figure 2, Figure 3.).

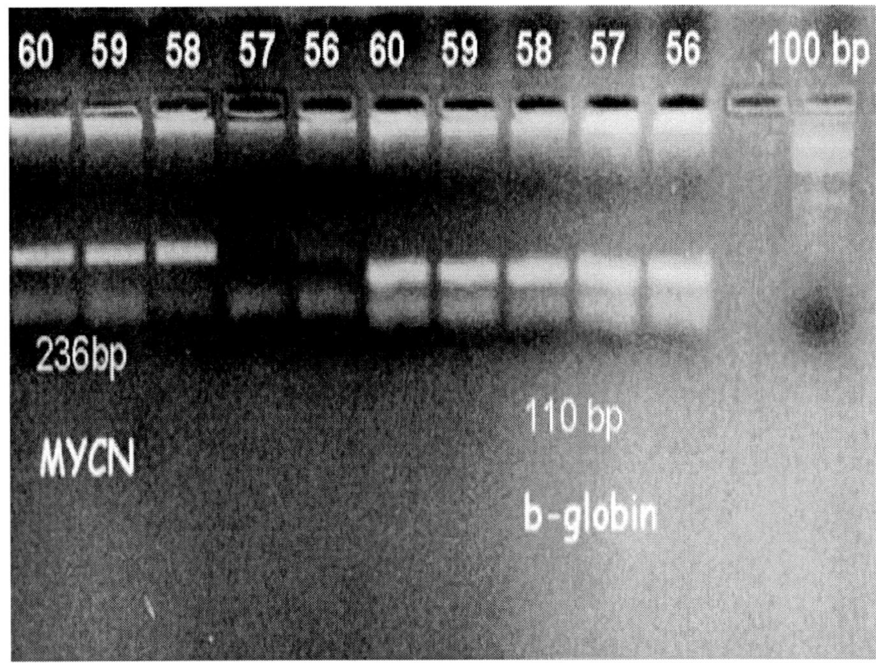

Figure 1. The PCR conditions for MYCN and b-globin amplification. Optimum conditions for both genes were 58-60°C. PCR cycles include: 1 x at 95 °C 5 min for initial denaturation, 30 x 94oC 1.15 min denaturation, 56-60°C 2 min annealing, 72°C 1.30 min extension, and 1 x 72°C 5 min final extension. The PCR products were electophoresed in 2% agarose.

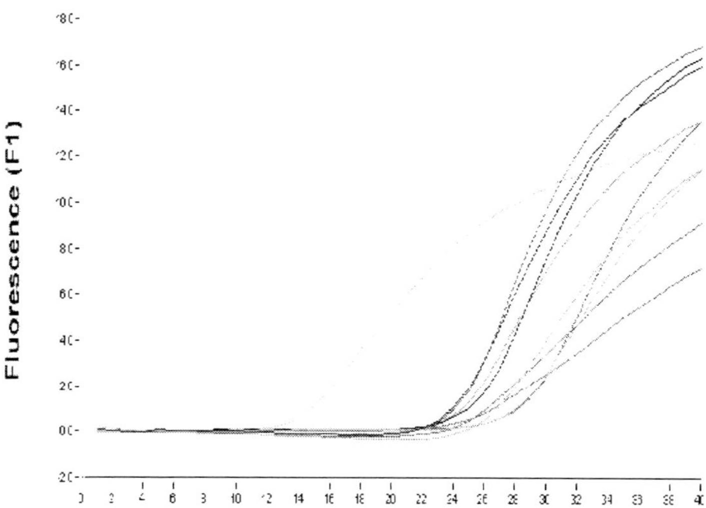

Figure 2. Preliminary results for the method of Real time PCR using the SYBR Green format. (90 ng of DNA were used /reaction). Y-axis shows the fluorescence detected while X-axis shows the cycle number. All the controls and samples show normal MYCN and b-globin copy status (enter the log phase of the reaction at 22 cycles). Kelly DNA shows amplified MYCN status (enters log phase at 13 cycles).

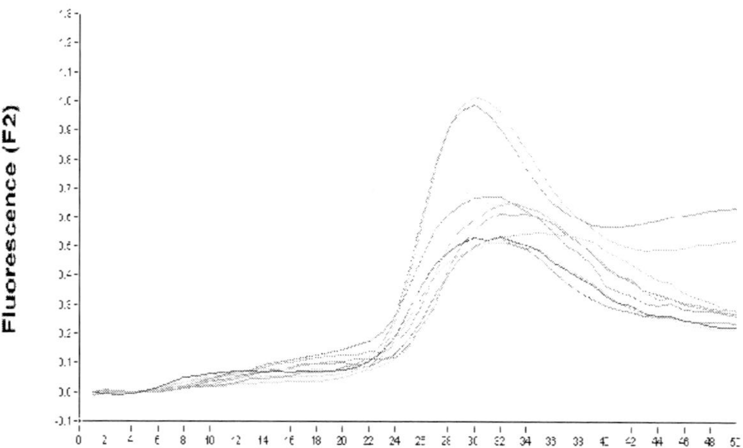

Figure 3. Preliminary results for the method of Real Time PCR using the Hyprobes format. (120 ng of DNA were used /reaction). Y-axis shows the fluorescence detected while X-axis shows the cycle number. Again all the controls and samples show normal MYCN and b-globin copy status (enter the log phase of the reaction at 21 cycles). Kelly DNA shows amplified MYCN status (enters log phase at 15 cycles).

Gene and Protein Microarray Analysis

Gene expression analysis plays an increasingly important role in many areas of biological research. Two recently developed methods for measurement of transcript abundance have gained much popularity and are frequently applied. Expression microarrays allow the parallel analysis of thousands of genes in two differentially labeled cDNA samples [54, 55], while reverse transcriptase Q-PCR provides quantitative analysis of expressed genes. In contrast to Q-PCR, cDNA microarray experiments require large amounts of good quality RNA (20–200 μg). Therefore, it is necessary to include an RNA amplification step following RNA extraction.

DNA microarray techniques have matured the furthest and currently the two most dominant types of platforms (biochips), are the oligonucleotide arrays and the spotted cDNA arrays. The technology is based on the principle that gene expression can be monitored indirectly by monitoring the amount of mRNA transcriptome present. For each gene a certain amount of mRNA transcript is produced in each cell. This mRNA is collected and reversely transcribed to DNA, using the RT-PCR method. The cDNA produced is hybridized to the oligonucleotide sequences or the cDNA sequences spotted on the biochip. DNA biochips have been used in cancer in order to define tumor markers for prognosis or diagnosis, predict clinical outcome, to classify tumors etc [56]. Gene expression profiles of 14 neuroblastoma tumors on cDNA microarrays consisting of 24,040 genes revealed 78 genes with mRNA expression levels significantly different between differentiating and poorly differentiated tumors. Genes associated with cell maturation and apoptosis were included in these, while 15 of them (cell adhesion molecules and cytoskeletal proteins), were overexpressed in stage 4 tumors [57]. In another study 99 genes were up regulated (overexpressed) and 24 genes were down regulated (underexpressed) compared to controls upon stimulation of neuroblastoma cells with the growth factor macrophage inhibitor factor (MIF). These genes included oncogenes, growth related genes, tumor metastatic genes and immuno-related genes [58].

cDNA microarrays have provided us with a huge amount of information regarding the transcriptional status of thousands of genes. But transcription is followed by translation and post-translational modifications (PTMs) and therefore the level or mRNA does not allow someone to predict the level of protein expression. This is partly due to the PTMs and partly due to the fact that protein maturation and degradation are dynamic processes, which can dramatically alter the final amount of active protein independently of the mRNA level [59].

The importance of protein, peptide and ligand arrays lies in the fact that in the near future whole proteome array chips, diagnostic chips and ligand chips will be readily available for prognostic and diagnostic purposes. Unlike cDNA microarrays where the hybridization of linear DNA or RNA is involved, protein-protein interactions depend on folded three-dimensional amino acid sequences. Therefore a number of problems arise with regards to maintaining the folded properties of the proteins and at the same time minimizing nonspecific binding [56]. The aim of the protein chips is the immobilization of the target molecule by the capture molecule, with the minimal non-specific binding possible, followed by its identification [59].

Most protein array technologies rely on spotting either the antigen (Ag) or the antibody (Ab) on derivatised glass surfaces using high precision robotic arrayers. These chips are then probed with fluorescently labelled purified proteins, antibodies, cell lysates or sera. Among the applications of antigen arrays is the ability to look for humoral response to various extrinsic proteins or tumor markers in sera [56].

The development, progression and invasiveness of cancer are processes governed by changes in protein levels or activities. Therefore the development of antibody arrays would prove a great tool for the early detection of these changes. In this case the Ab is spotted on the slide while the cell lysate, sera or purified protein is labelled fluorescently and probed on the slide [56,60].

Several technical aspects of protein microarray chips need to be considered since there is no simple method for protein amplification such as PCR for the cDNA microarrays. Proteins are much more complex molecules than DNA or mRNA, therefore one cannot define protein detection and immobilisation strategies that do not discriminate against other proteins. They can easily lose their biochemical activity due to denaturation, dehydration or oxidation, while approximately 50% are insoluble and of an unstable structure. Finally, Ab-Ag interactions are characterised by broad specificity and affinity making it difficult for specific detection [60].

The concept of protein-expression microarrays that yield definitive data for any protein expression of a chosen sample has the potential to handle large number of samples while providing a high degree of proteomic coverage following differential protein expression in multiple tissue and cell types for each patient.

Essential requirement in the construction of such protein arrays will be the parallel generation and screening of large-repertoire libraries of recognition molecules. The application of techniques for immobilization of these recognition molecules on suitable surface chemistries is another important factor. Other requirements include the tagging of proteins (stoichiometrically), so that their ability to bind specifically is not influenced, sensitive systems for the detection of the bound target protein and bio-computing [61,62]. These techniques will have to be mutually compatible. Immobilization of the arrayed recognition molecules in a site-directed manner so that their specificity is preserved may prove more difficult to achieve than with DNA arrays [63]. Imperative for all antibody-based technologies is to overcome limitations in availability, size and quality of the recognition molecule (antibody) library. The libraries available today limit the use of antibody microarrays as a proteomics tool in the original holistic sense and favor more specific diagnostic applications targeting a small number of known diagnostic marker proteins [64].

Proteomic Markers in Neuroblastoma

Tumor markers are biomolecules needed for screening, diagnosis, staging, prognosis, monitoring treatment response, or detection of tumor recurrence. The ideal tumor marker should be highly specific for a single type of tumor, and not related to any other pathological conditions. Tumor markers that are expressed in cells during embryological development and cancer cells are relatively specific to tumor cells, but not to the cancer type. Another type of tumor markers are those which may be overexpressed in tumor cells but are also expressed moderately in normal tissues.

A versatile tumor marker should be easily detected by simple clinical chemistry or immunoassay. The tumor cells release some markers to the blood stream, whereas others are only detected on the tissue sections. The former is of more practical benefit, as the methods of detection are less invasive and only a blood sample is needed. If a marker can only be detected on tissue sections, its clinical use, especially for screening or early diagnosis, is limited. The ideal tumor marker for diagnosis or screening should be detectable in biological fluids before the tumor can be visualized by imaging, thereby permitting treatment at a curative stage.

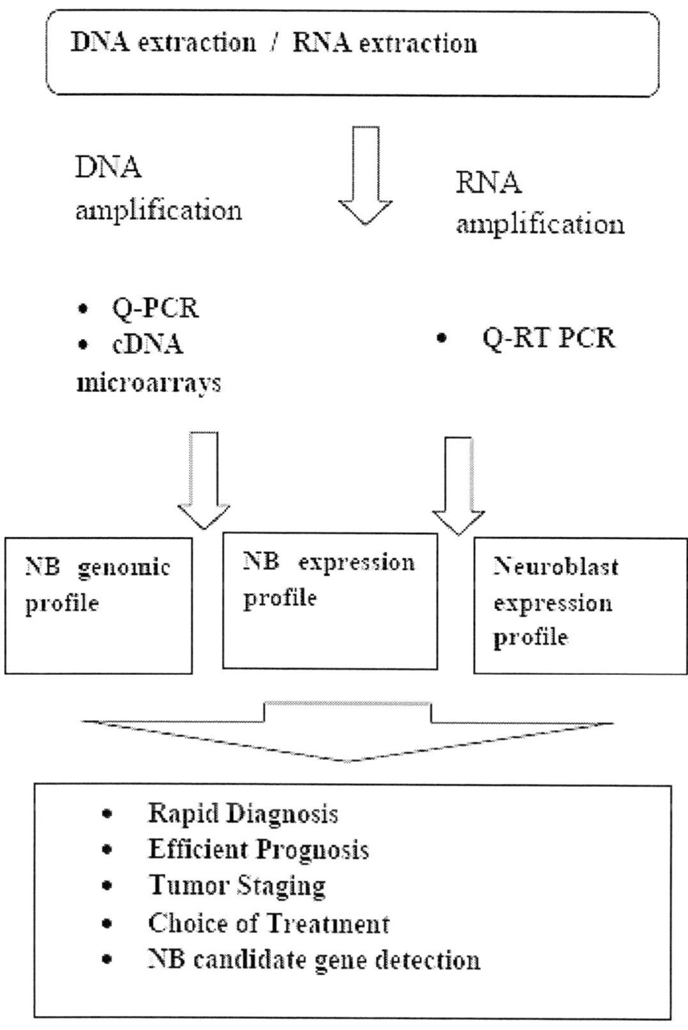

Figure 4. Genome and proteome profiling will lead to improved diagnosis and prediction of patient outcome, and will help the identification of relevant tumor candidate genes.

Neuroblastomas are considered to be embryonal tumors, which means that they originate as a result of a developmental defect during the normal differentiation from progenitor cells to mature tissue cells. The molecular pathways implicated in the normal development of the neuro-endocrine cells should have an important role in the progression of the disease (Table 1). Therefore profiling of the protein molecules implicated in the progression of the disease would be appropriate in order to identify proteomic markers that could be used in the diagnosis or the prognosis of the disease.

Neurotrophins are important soluble factors that regulate growth, development, survival and repair of the nervous system. They use two classes of receptors for their signalling pathways, the Trk tyrosine kinase receptors and the p75 neurotrophin receptor ($p75^{NTR}$). The receptors TrkA, TrkB and TrkC can bind the nerve growth factor (NGF), brain-derived neurotrophic factor (BDNF) and neurotrophin-3 (NT-3), respectively, while neurotrophin-4/5 (NT-4/5) binds to TrkB and weakly to TrkA. $p75^{NTR}$ is a low-affinity receptor and member of the tumor necrosis factor (TNF) receptor super family and can bind all four neurotrophins [65,66].

Trka ,Trkb and Trkc Expression in Neuroblastoma

High expression of the high-affinity receptor TrkA is found in mature sympathetic ganglia as well as in tumors with favorable prognosis. High TrkA expression is associated with younger age, lower stage and absence of MYCN amplification. Vice versa, low TrkA expression is associated with a poor prognosis and MYCN amplification. In the absence of NGF, TrkA expression will lead to apoptosis, while binding of NGF increases cell survival and differentiation of neuroblasts [66,67]. Schwann cells, which can be part of the stromal environment of the neuroblasts, are a known source of NGF production [68]. Increase of stromal components in neuroblastoma tumors is also associated with a better prognosis and cellular differentiation [69]. The absence of NGF in the microenvironment of tumors may play a role in the regression of neuroblastomas seen in individual patients, especially infants.

Another possible connection of TrkA to regression of neuroblastoma tumors is formed by the oncogene HRAS (ras family of genes). Increased HRAS expression is a favorable predictor of outcome in neuroblastomas and strongly correlated to high expression of TrkA. In neuroblastoma cell lines, overexpression of wild-type HRAS protein caused the cells to undergo apoptosis, whereas overexpression of a mutant HRAS did not. The expression of the HRAS coupled with high TrkA expression can induce caspase-independent cell death in neuroblastoma cell lines and may play a role in the spontaneous regression of neuroblastomas [70].

The activation of $p75^{NTR}$ leads to increased apoptosis in neuroblasts. High expression of $p75^{NTR}$ is more pronounced in lower-risk neuroblastomas, whereas MYCN amplification is strongly associated with low expression of $p75^{NTR}$ [71-73].

High expression of TrkB is preferentially found in high-risk tumors, particularly in those with amplification of MYCN [74]. There is evidence that TrkB and TrkC are expressed in the earlier development of the ganglion cells of the sympathetic nervous system, which will switch to mainly TrkA expression in the mature ganglion cell [75]. The maturation arrest of cells with high expression of TrkB seems to occur at an earlier stage of neuroblast development than these with high TrkA expression. TrkC expression is, like TrkA, predominantly found in lower stage, MYCN single copy tumors.

Table 1. Genetic and molecular characteristics of neuroblastomas LOH, loss of heterozygosity; Trk, tyrosine receptor kinase; CCND1, gene for cyclin-D1

Characteristic	Genetic/Molecular Defect	Prognosis
Ploidy	Amplified MYCN	Poor
LOH 1p	Amplified MYCN	Poor
LOH 2q	Loss of Caspase 8 /	Poor
LOH 3p	amplified MYCN	Intermediate
TrkA	LOH 11q.14q /	Good
overexpression	MYCN normal	Poor
TrkB	HRAS	Good
overexpression	overexpression	Good
TrkC	Ploidy, amplified	?
overexpression	MYCN	
P75NTR	?	
overexpression	?	
CCND1	CCND1	
overexpression	amplification	

MYCN Protein Expression and Apoptosis in Neuroblastoma

Many observations have shown that MYCN and its family member c-MYC can induce apoptosis [75, 76]. The apoptotic properties of c-MYC have been studied in more detail than for MYCN, and several data to support a role for MYCN in apoptosis are based on studies with c-MYC. However, all the available data suggest that MYCN and c-MYC have similar functions, but in different cell types. In fact, it was even shown that MYCN could functionally replace c-MYC in murine development [77].

Initially, it was shown that apoptosis could be induced in fibroblasts with ectopic expression of c-MYC if cultured in the absence of sufficient survival factors [78]. A widely supported interpretation of these and similar observations about the apoptotic potential of oncogenes is that the induction of the cell cycle after expression of oncogenes also sensitises cells to apoptosis. Apoptosis, however, will be suppressed as long as appropriate survival factors are available for proliferation and growth. This suggests a coupling between the cell cycle and apoptosis and implies that cells with oncogenic mutations can only outgrow their paracrine environment in the presence of sufficient growth factors, or if apoptosis is inhibited. Examples of inhibition of apoptosis in combination with up-regulation of the cell cycle are common in carcinogenesis. In fact, in the majority of all cancer types, a combined loss of TP53 and activation of oncogenes like c-MYC or RAS can be found. In particular, for c-MYC, it was shown that in normal, mature cells activation of c-MYC induces uniform cell proliferation, accompanied by overwhelming apoptosis that rapidly erodes cell mass. However, upon induced co-expression of BCL-XL, c-MYC triggered rapid and uniform progression into invasive tumors. Subsequent c-MYC deactivation induced rapid regression associated with vascular degeneration and cell apoptosis [79].

It seems that in neuroblastomas a similar interplay between cell growth and apoptosis exists involving MYCN. It has been convincingly shown that exogenous overexpression of MYCN sensitises neuroblastoma cell lines to many apoptotic triggers, such as γ-IFN, TRAIL, FasL, but also to exogenous stimuli like doxorubicin [75,76]. Neuroblastomas that overexpress MYCN protein, do not apoptose spontaneously or after stimulation. This is considered to result from overexpression of BCL2 or BCL-XL in neuroblastomas. Increased levels of BCL2 can counteract the MYCN induced activation of BAX. Overexpression of BCL2 or BCL-XL has been observed in high-risk neuroblastomas with amplified MYCN. Incomplete or ineffective apoptosis is a basic defect in these tumors [80]. Also, the overexpression of both BCL2 and BCL-XL was able to block apoptosis induced by various chemotherapeutic agents, like cisplatin, doxorubicin, etoposide and betulinic acid. Therefore, it was suggested that the observed expression of these proteins in tumors might contribute to the drug resistance, characteristic of high-risk neuroblastomas [81]. It should be stressed however, that structural alterations of the BCL2 and BCL-X_L genes, or any of the other genes involved in the intrinsic apoptotic pathway have never been shown [39,82].

The caspase 8-dependent pathway (CASP 8) is an essential pathway in neuro-endocrine development and blocking of this route is important in the pathogenesis of aggressive neuroendocrine tumors. The role of MYCN in the extrinsic apoptotic route is not very clear, although the down-regulation of CASP 8 in neuroblastomas seems closely connected to overexpression of MYCN. However, a direct influence of MYCN on CASP 8 has not been shown, since the overexpression of MYCN protein does not induce CASP 8 hypermethylation or down-regulation [76,82,83].

NM23-H1 and NM23-H2 Protein Expression in Neuroblastoma

NM23H1 is a highly interesting candidate gene for an important role in neuroblastoma pathogenesis, associated with gain of chromosome 17q. The NM23H1 gene maps at the short arm of chromosome 17 (17q22), i.e. just within the common amplified region of 17q. NM23H1 was originally described as a suppressor of metastasis with low or absent expression in mainly breast cancer and melanoma. In several other malignancies, NM23H1 acts as an oncogene and increased serum levels of NM23H1 protein correlated with poor prognosis and increased aggressivenes, as is the case in neuroblastoma [84]. Interestingly, NM23H1 is part of a gene family, which includes also NM23H2, another gene that colocalizes at 17q22. NM23H1 and NM23H2 are both up regulated by MYCN and c-MYC in neuroblastoma. Therefore amplification of MYCN in tumors with a gain of 17q will lead to a synergistic accumulation of the NM23H1 and NM23H2 mRNA levels. It seems that the protein NM23H2 (but not NM23H1) is involved in chemotherapy resistance in neuroblastomas with 17q gain (has an anti-apoptotic effect) [84].

TP53, TP73 and Deltanp73 Protein Expression in Neuroblastoma

The nuclear phosphoprotein TP53 plays a central role in the pathogenesis of human cancers. TP53 is a checkpoint protein for the cell cycle and monitors DNA damage. Activation of TP53 will lead to cell cycle arrest or apoptosis. Defects in the p53 gene play a role in more than 50% of all human neoplasias. It usually concerns LOH of one allele, in combination with a missense point mutation. In neuroblastomas, p53 is rarely mutated [85]. However, it has also been shown that the TP53 protein is functionally inactivated through sequestration in the cytoplasm in undifferentiated neuroblastomas [86]. Recently, a cytoplasmic protein Parc was identified, responsible for cytoplasmic sequestration of ectopic TP53 [87].

The p73 gene is a structural homologue of p53, located at chromosome 1p36.3 [88] and TP73 protein induces apoptosis similar to TP53. p73 maps within the SRO of 1p deletion in neuroblastomas therefore it appeared to be a good candidate tumor suppressor gene. So far, mutations of p73 have not been found, except in malignant lymphomas, where the inactivation of p73 has been observed as a result of bi-allelic hypermethylation [89].

Recently, a truncated anti-apoptotic isoform, DeltaNp73, which antagonizes both TP53 and the full-length TP73 protein, has gained attention. So far, expression of this variant in neuroblastoma patients significantly correlated with age at diagnosis, urinary excretion of catecholamine-derivatives, and reduced survival. The role of this protein needs further investigation in larger cohorts to establish its role in the pathogenesis of neuroblastomas [90].

Cyclin D1

Genetic aberrations and overexpression of cyclin D1 (CCND1) have been identified for several human neoplasms, such as mantle cell lymphoma, head and neck squamous cell carcinoma, lung cancer and breast cancer. D-type cyclins play an essential role in cell cycle progression, as they control cyclin-dependent kinases (CDKs). Recently, very high expression of CCND1 RNA and protein levels was found in approximately two-thirds of cell lines and tumors. In addition, amplification of the CCND1 gene was found in one neuroblastoma cell line and 4 neuroblastoma tumors [91]. There was no obvious relation to prognostic factors, such as amplification of MYCN, age, stage or any other factor. It suggests that CCND1 is a frequently overexpressed oncogene in neuroblastomas.

Conclusion

Genomics has provided a vast amount of information linking gene activity with disease. It is now recognized, however, that there are a number of reasons why gene sequence information and the pattern of gene activity in a cell do not provide a complete and accurate profile of a protein's abundance or its final structure and state of activity. After transcription from DNA to RNA, the gene transcript can be spliced in different ways prior to translation into protein. Following translation, most proteins are chemically changed through post-translational modification, mainly through the addition of carbohydrate and phosphate groups. Such modification plays a vital role in modulating the function of many proteins but is not directly coded by genes. As a consequence, the information from a single gene can encode as many as 50 different protein species. Therefore genomic information often does not provide an accurate profile of protein abundance, structure and activity. Since it is proteins and, to a much lesser extent, other types of biological molecules that are directly involved in both normal and disease-associated biochemical processes, a more complete understanding of disease may be gained by looking directly at the proteins present within a diseased cell or tissue and this is achieved through the proteome and proteomics.

Proteomics is a scientific discipline, which detects proteins that are associated with a disease by means of their altered levels of expression between control and disease states. It enables correlations to be drawn between the range of proteins produced by a cell or tissue and the initiation or progression of a disease state.

Proteins are far more complex than DNA on many levels. DNA consists of just four basic building blocks: adenine, guanine, cytosine and thymine [A, G, C, T]. Various combinations of 20 different amino acids make up human proteins. The order in which As, Cs, Gs and Ts string together gives scientists the key to everything there is to know about genes, most of which have the same function: coding for proteins. In contrast, the three-dimensional shapes of proteins determine their functions, which seem endless. Proteins provide the structure of all cells and allow them to move around. They make up the messengers that constantly traffic between immune-system cells and they control the firing of neurotransmitters that allows us to think, the contraction of muscles that allows us to move, and the very on/off switches in our genes that allow us to make even more proteins. Proteins blow genes out of the water in sheer numbers, too. The Human Genome Project found between 30,000 and 40,000 genes scattered throughout our chromosomes potentially encoding 40,000 different proteins. Alternative RNA splicing and post-translational modification may increase this number to 2 million proteins or protein fragments.

Recent developments in protein microarray technology provide a versatile tool to study protein-protein, protein-nucleic acid, protein-lipid, enzyme-substrate, and protein-drug interactions. Other types of microarrays, though not fully developed, also show great potential in diagnostics, protein profiling, and drug identification and validation.

Proteome research permits the discovery of new protein markers for diagnostic purposes and of novel molecular targets for drug discovery. The abundance of information provided by proteome research is entirely complementary with the genetic information being generated by genomic research. Proteomics will make a key contribution to the development of functional genomics. The combination of proteomics and genomics will play a major role in biomedical research and will have a significant impact on the development of the diagnostic and therapeutic products of the future.

References

[1] Brodeur G.M, J. Pritchard, F. Berthold, N.L. Carlsen, V. Castel, R.P. Castelberry, B. De Bernardi, A.E. Evans, M. Favrot, F. Hedborg et al. Revisions of the international criteria for neuroblastoma diagnosis, staging, and response to treatment. *J. Clin. Oncol.* 1993; 11:1466–1477.

[2] Hayes FA, Green A, Hustu HO, et al. Surgicopathologic staging of neuroblastoma prognostic significance of regional lymph node metastases. *J. Pediatr.* 1983; 102:59-62.

[3] Cotterill SJ, Pearson AD, Pritchard J, et al. Clinical prognostic factors in 1277 patients with neuroblastoma: results of The European Neuroblastoma Study Group 'Survey' 1982-1992. *Eur. J. Cancer* 2000 ; 36:901-8.

[4] Bowman LC, Hancock ML, Santana VM, et al. Impact of intensified therapy on clinical outcome in infants and children with neuroblastoma: the St Jude Children's Research Hospital experience, 1962 to 1988. *J. Clin. Oncol.* 1991; 9:1599-608.

[5] Look AT, Hayes FA, Shuster JJ, et al. Clinical relevance of tumor cell ploidy and Nmyc gene amplification in childhood neuroblastoma: a Pediatric Oncology Group study. *J. Clin. Oncol.* 1991; 9:581-91.

[6] Schmidt ML, Lukens JN, Seeger RC, et al. Biologic factors determine prognosis in infants with stage IV neuroblastoma: A prospective Children's Cancer Group study. *J. Clin. Oncol.* 2000; 18:1260-8.

[7] Berthold F, Trechow R, Utsch S, et al. Prognostic factors in metastatic neuroblastoma. A multivariate analysis of 182 cases. *Am. J. Pediatr Hematol. Oncol.* 1992; 14:207-15.

[8] Matthay KK, Perez C, Seeger RC, et al. Successful treatment of stage III neuroblastoma based on prospective biologic staging: a Children's Cancer Group study. *J. Clin. Oncol.* 1998; 16:1256-64.

[9] Ladenstein R, Ambros IM, Pötschger U, et al. Prognostic significance of DNA ditetraploidy in neuroblastoma. *Med. Pediatr. Oncol.* 2001; 36:83-92.

[10] Look A.T., F.A. Hayes, J.J. Shuster, E.C. Douglass, R.P. Castleberry, L.C. Bowman, E.I. Smith and G.M. Brodeur et al. Clinical relevance of tumor cell ploidy and N-myc gene amplification in childhood neuroblastoma: a Pediatric Oncology Group study. *J. Clin. Oncol.* 1991; 9:581–591.

[11] Brinkley B.R. Managing the centrosome numbers game: from chaos to stability in cancer cell division. *Trends Cell Biol.* 2001; 11:18–21.

[12] Tonini GP, Boni L, Pession A, et al. MYCN oncogene amplification in neuroblastoma is associated with worse prognosis, except in stage 4s: the Italian experience with 295 children. *J. Clin. Oncol.* 1997; 15: 85-93.

[13] Bown N, Lastowska M, Cotterill S, et al. 17q gain in neuroblastoma predicts adverse clinical outcome. U.K. Cancer Cytogenetics Group and the U.K. Children's Cancer Study Group. *Med. Pediatr. Oncol.* 2001; 36:14-9.

[14] Bown N, Cotterill S, Lastowska M, et al. Gain of chromosome arm 17q and adverse outcome in patients with neuroblastoma. *N. Engl. J. Med.* 1999; 340:1954-61.

[15] Krams M, Hero B, Berthold F, et al. Proliferation marker KI-S5 discriminates between favorable and adverse prognosis in advanced stages of neuroblastoma with and without MYCN amplification. *Cancer* 2002; 94:854-61.

[16] Spieker N., M. Beitsma, P. Van Sluis, A. Chan, H. Caron and R. Versteeg . Three chromosomal rearrangements in neuroblastoma cluster within a 300-kb region on 1p36.1. *Genes Chromosomes Cancer* 2001; 31:172–181.

[17] Bauer A., L. Savelyeva, A. Claas, C. Praml, F. Berthold and M. Schwab. Smallest region of overlapping deletion in 1p36 in human neuroblastoma: a 1 Mbp cosmid and PAC contig. *Genes Chromosomes Cancer* 2001; 31:228–239.

[18] White P.S., P.M. Thompson, B.A. Seifried, E.P. Sulman, S.J. Jensen, C. Guo, J.M. Maris, M.D. Hogarty, C. Allen, J.A. Biegel, T.C. Matise, S.G. Gregory, C.P. Reynolds and G.M. Brodeur. Detailed molecular analysis of 1p36 in neuroblastoma. *Med. Pediatr. Oncol.* 2001; 36:37–41.

[19] Nakagawara A, Arima-Nakagawara M, Scavarda NJ, et al. Association between high levels of expression of the TRK gene and favorable outcome in human neuroblastoma. *N. Engl. J. Med.* 1993; 328:847-54.

[20] Poremba C, Hero B, Goertz HG, et al. Traditional and emerging molecular markers in neuroblastoma prognosis: the good, the bad and the ugly. *Klin Padiatr* 2001; 213:18690.

[21] Hann HW, Evans AE, Siegel SE, et al. Prognostic importance of serum ferritin in patients with Stages III and IV neuroblastoma: the Childrens Cancer Study Group experience. *Cancer Res.* 1985; 45:2843-8.

[22] Shuster JJ, McWilliams NB, Castleberry R, et al. Serum lactate dehydrogenase in childhood neuroblastoma. A Pediatric Oncology Group recursive partitioning study. *Am. J. Clin. Oncol.* 1992;15:295-303.

[23] Massaron S, Seregni E, Luksch R, et al. Neuron-specific enolase evaluation in patients with neuroblastoma. *Tumour Biol.* 1998; 19:261-8.

[24] De Bernardi B, Pianca C, Boni L, et al. Disseminated neuroblastoma (stage IV and IVS) in the first year of life. Outcome related to age and stage. Italian Cooperative Group on Neuroblastoma. *Cancer* 1992; 70:1625-33.

[25] Combaret V, Gross N, Lasset C, et al. Clinical relevance of CD44 cell-surface expression and N-myc gene amplification in a multicentric analysis of 121 pediatric neuroblastomas. *J. Clin. Oncol.* 1996; 14:25-34.

[26] Reynolds CP, Seeger RC. Detection of minimal residual disease in bone marrow during or after therapy as a prognostic marker for high-risk neuroblastoma. *J. Pediatr. Hematol. Oncol.* 2001; 23:150-2.

[27] Burchill SA, Lewis IJ, Abrams KR, et al. Circulating neuroblastoma cells detected by reverse transcriptase polymerase chain reaction for tyrosine hydroxylase mRNA are an independent poor prognostic indicator in stage 4 neuroblastoma in children over 1 year. *J. Clin. Oncol.* 2001; 19:1795-801.

[28] Seeger RC, Reynolds CP, Gallego R, et al. Quantitative tumor cell content of bone marrow and blood as a predictor of outcome in stage IV neuroblastoma: a Children's Cancer Group Study. *J. Clin. Oncol.* 2000; 18:4067-76.

[29] [29] Caron H., P. van Sluis, J. de Kraker, J. Bokkerink, M. Egeler, G. Laureys, R. Slater, A. Westerveld, P.A. Voute and R. Versteeg. Allelic loss

of chromosome 1p as a predictor of unfavourable outcome in patients with neuroblastoma. *N. Engl. J. Med.* 1996; 334:225– 230.

[30] Maris JM, Matthay KK. Molecular biology of neuroblastoma. *J. Clin. Oncol.* 1999; 17:2264-79.

[31] Lastowska M, Cullinane C, Variend S, et al. Comprehensive genetic and histopathologic study reveals three types of neuroblastoma tumors. *J. Clin. Oncol.* 2001; 19:3080-90.

[32] Reynolds CP. Ras and Seppuku in neuroblastoma. *J. Natl. Cancer Inst.* 2002; 94:319-21.

[33] Hiyama E, Hiyama K, Yokoyama T, et al. Correlating telomerase activity levels with human neuroblastoma outcomes. *Nat. Med.* 1995; 1:249-55.

[34] Hiyama E, Reynolds CP. Telomerase as a biological and prognostic marker in neuroblastoma. In: Brodeur GM, Sawada T, Tsuchida Y: Neuroblastoma. New York, NY: Elsevier Science, 2000, pp 159-174.

[35] Kitanaka C, Kato K, Ijiri R, et al. Increased Ras expression and caspase-independent neuroblastoma cell death: possible mechanism of spontaneous neuroblastoma regression. *J. Natl. Cancer Inst.* 2002; 94:358-68.

[36] Yamamoto K, Ohta S, Ito E, et al. Marginal decrease in mortality and marked increase in incidence as a result of neuroblastoma screening at 6 months of age: cohort study in seven prefectures in Japan. *J. Clin. Oncol.* 2002; 20:1209-14.

[37] S. Solinas-Toldo, S. Lampel, S. Stilgenbauer, J. Nickolenko, A. Benner, H. Dohner, T. Cremer, P. Lichter. Matrix-based comparative genomic hybridization: biochips to screen for genomic imbalances, *Genes Chromosomes Cancer* 1997; 20: 399–407.

[38] D. Pinkel, R. Segraves, D. Sudar, S. Clark, I. Poole, D. Kowbel, C. Collins, W.L. Kuo, C. Chen, Y. Zhai, S.H. Dairkee, B.M. Ljung, J.W. Gray, D.G. Albertson. High resolution analysis of DNA copy number variation using comparative genomic hybridization to microarrays, *Nat. Genet.* 1998; 20:207–211.

[39] M. Schena, D. Shalon, R.W. Davis, P.O. Brown. Quantitative monitoring of gene expression patterns with a complementary DNA microarray. *Science* 1995; 270:467– 470.

[40] D.J. Lockhart, H. Dong, M.C. Byrne, M.T. Follettie, M.V. Gallo, M.S. Chee, M. Mittmann, C. Wang, M. Kobayashi, H. Horton, E.L. Brown. Expression monitoring by hybridization to high-density oligonucleotide arrays. *Nat. Biotechnol.* 1996; 14:1675– 1680.

[41] Bustin S.A.. Absolute quantification of mRNA using real-time reverse transcription polymerase chain reaction assays. *J. Mol. Endocrinol.* 2000; 25:169–193.

[42] Wilkins M.R., J.-C. Sanchez, A.A. Gooley, R.D. Appel, I. Humphrey-Smith, D.F. Hochstrasser and K.L. Williams. Progress with proteome projects: why all proteins expressed by a genome should be identified and how to do it. *Biotechnol. Genet Eng. Rev.* 1996; 13:19–50.

[43] Maris JM, Weiss MJ, Guo C, et al. Loss of heterozygosity at 1p36 independently predicts for disease progression but not decreased overall survival probability in neuroblastoma patients: a Children's Cancer Group study. *J. Clin. Oncol.* 2000; 18: 188899.

[44] Cohn SL, London WB, Huang D, et al. MYCN expression is not prognostic of adverse outcome in advanced-stage neuroblastoma with nonamplified MYCN. *J. Clin. Oncol.* 2000; 18:3604-13.

[45] Schwab M., H.E. Varmus and J.M. Bishop. Human N-myc gene contributes to neoplastic transformation of mammalian cells in culture. *Nature* 1985; 316:160–162.

[46] Small M.B., N. Hay, M. Schwab and J.M. Bishop. Neoplastic transformation by the human gene N-myc. *Mol. Cell Biol.* 1987; 7:1638–1645.

[47] Weiss W.A., K. Aldape, G. Mohapatra, B.G. Feuerstein and J.M. Bishop. Targeted expression of MYCN causes neuroblastoma in transgenic mice. *EMBO J.* 1997; 16:2985–2995.

[48] Schmidt M.L, H.R. Salwen, C.F. Manohar, N. Ikegaki and S.L. Cohn. The biological effects of antisense N-myc expression in human neuroblastoma. *Cell Growth Differ.* 1994; 5:171–178.

[49] Sato Y., Kobayashi Y., Sasaki H., Toyama T., Kondo S., Kiriyama M. and Fujii Y. Expression of ID2 mRNA in neuroblastoma and normal ganglion. *Eur. J. Surg. Oncol.* 2003; 29:284-7.

[50] Strieder V, Lutz W. Regulation of N-myc expression in development and disease. *Cancer Lett.* 2002; 180:107-19.

[51] Walker C, Joyce KA, Thompson_Hehir J, Davies MP, Gibbs FE, Halliwell N, Lloyd BH, Machell Y, Roebuck MM, Salisbury J, Sibson DR, Du Plessis D, Broome J, Rossi ML. Characterisation of molecular alterations in microdissected archival gliomas. *Acta Neuropathol* (Berl) 2001; 101:321-33.

[52] Noguera R, Canete A, Pellin A, Ruiz A, Tasso M, Navarro S, Castel V, Llombart_Bosch A. MYCN gain and MYCN amplification in a stage 4S neuroblastoma. *Cancer Genet. Cytogenet.* 2003; 140:157-61.

[53] Combaret V, Audoynaud C, Iacono I, Favrot MC, Schell M, Bergeron C, Puisieux Circulating MYCN DNA as a tumor-specific marker in neuroblastoma patients. *Cancer Res.* 2002; 62:3646-8.

[54] Caron H., P. van Sluis, J. de Kraker, J. Bokkerink, M. Egeler, G. Laureys, R. Slater, A. Westerveld, P.A. Voute and R. Versteeg. Allelic loss of chromosome 1p as a predictor of unfavorable outcome in patients with neuroblastoma. *N. Engl. J. Med.* 1996; 334: 225– 230.

[55] Spieker N., M. Beitsma, P. Van Sluis, A. Chan, H. Caron and R. Versteeg. Three chromosomal rearrangements in neuroblastoma cluster within a 300-kb region on 1p36.1. *Genes Chromosomes Cancer* 2001; 31:172–181.

[56] Sreekumar A, Chinnaiyan AM. Protein microarrays: a powerful tool to study cancer. *Curr. Opin. Mol. Ther.* 2002; 4:587-93.

[57] Yamanaka Y, Hamazaki Y, Sato Y, Ito K, Watanabe K, Heike T, Nakahata T, Nakamura Y. Maturational sequence of neuroblastoma revealed by molecular analysis on cDNA microarrays. *Int. J. Oncol.* 2002; 21:803-7.

[58] Fan J, Tam P, Woude GV, Ren Y. Normalization and analysis of cDNA microarrays using within-array replications applied to neuroblastoma cell response to a cytokine. *Proc. Natl. Acad. Sci. USA* 2004; 101:1135-40.

[59] Peter J. Chips for proteomics or just hype?. *Bio. Techniques* 2002; 33:S4-S13.

[60] Kusnezow W, Jacob A, Walijew A, Diehl F, Hoheisel JD. Antibody microarrays: an evaluation of production parameters. *Proteomics* 2003; 3:254-64.

[61] Figeys D. and D. Pinto. Proteomics on a chip: promising developments. *Electrophoresis* 2001; 22:208–216.

[62] R.E. Jenkins and S.R. Pennington. Arrays for protein expression profiling: towards a viable alternative to two-dimensional gel electrophoresis?. *Proteomics* 2001; 1:13–29.

[63] Chemla Y.R., H.L. Grossman, Y. Poon, R. McDermott, R. Stevens, M.D. Alper and J. Clarke. Ultrasensitive magnetic biosensor for homogenous immunoassay. *Proc. Natl. Acad. Sci. USA* 2000; 97:14268–14272.

[64] RoweTaitt C.A., J.P. Golden, M.J. Feldstein, J.J. Cras, K.E. Hoffman and F.S. Ligler. Array biosensor for detection of biohazards. *Biosens Bioelectron* 2000; 14:785–794.

[65] Lee F.S., A.H. Kim, G. Khursigara and M.V. Chao. The uniqueness of being a neurotrophin receptor. *Curr. Opin. Neurobiol.* 2001; 11:281–286.

[66] Patapoutian A. and L.F. Reichardt. Trk receptors. mediators of neurotrophin action. *Curr. Opin. Neurobiol.* 2001; 11:272–280.

[67] Ambros PF, Brodeur GM. Concept of tumorigenesis and regression. In: Brodeur GM, Sawada T, Tsuchida Y: Neuroblastoma. New York, NY: Elsevier Science 2000, pp. 2132.

[68] Tanaka T., T. Sugimoto and T. Sawada. Prognostic discrimination among neuroblastomas according to Ha-ras/trk A gene expression. a comparison of the profiles of neuroblastomas detected clinically and those detected through mass screening. *Cancer* 1998; 83:1626–1633.

[69] Kitanaka C., K. Kato, R. Ijiri, K. Sakurada, A. Tomiyama, K. Noguchi, Y. Nagashima, Nakagawara, T. Momoi, Y. Toyoda, H. Kigasawa, T. Nishi, M. Shirouzu, S. Yokoyama, Y. Tanaka and Y. Kuchino. Increased Ras expression and caspaseindependent neuroblastoma cell death: possible mechanism of spontaneous neuroblastoma regression. *J. Natl. Cancer Inst.* 2002; 94:358–368.

[70] Eggert A., M.A. Grotzer, T.J. Zuzak, B.R. Wiewrodt, R. Ho, N. Ikegaki and G.M. Brodeur. Resistance to tumor necrosis factor-related apoptosis-inducing ligand (TRAIL)-induced apoptosis in neuroblastoma cells correlates with a loss of caspase-8 expression. *Cancer Res.* 2001; 61:1314–1319.

[71] Casaccia-Bonnefil P., B.D. Carter, R.T. Dobrowsky and M.V. Chao. Death of oligodendrocytes mediated by the interaction of nerve growth factor with its receptor p75. *Nature* 1996; 383:716–719.

[72] Nakagawara A., C.G. Azar, N.J. Scavarda and G.M. Brodeur. Expression and function of TRK-B and BDNF in human neuroblastomas. *Mol. Cell Biol.* 1994; 14:759–767.

[73] Birren S.J., L. Lo and D.J. Anderson. Sympathetic neuroblasts undergo a developmental switch in trophic dependence. *Development* 1993; 119:597–610.

[74] Melino G., M. Draoui, L. Bellincampi, F. Bernassola, S. Bernardini, M. Piacentini, U. Reichert and P. Cohen. Retinoic acid receptors alpha and

gamma mediate the induction of "tissue" transglutaminase activity and apoptosis in human neuroblastoma cells. *Exp. Cell Res.* 1997; 235:55–61.

[75] Fulda S., W. Lutz, M. Schwab and K.M. Debatin. MycN sensitizes neuroblastoma cells for drug-triggered apoptosis. *Med. Pediatr. Oncol.* 2000; 35:582–584.

[76] van Noesel M.M., K. Hahlen, F.G. Hakvoort-Cammel and R.M. Egeler. Neuroblastoma 4S: a heterogeneous disease with variable risk factors and treatment strategies. *Cancer* 1997; 80:834–843.

[77] Malynn B.A., I.M. de Alboran, R.C. O'Hagan, R. Bronson, L. Davidson, R.A. DePinho and F.W. Alt. N-myc can functionally replace c-myc in murine development, cellular growth, and differentiation. *Genes. Dev.* 2000; 14:1390–1399.

[78] Evan G.I., A.H. Wyllie, C.S. Gilbert, T.D. Littlewood, H. Land, M. Brooks, C.M. Waters, L.Z. Penn and D.C. Hancock. Induction of apoptosis in fibroblasts by c-myc protein. *Cell* 1992; 69: 119–128.

[79] Pelengaris S., M. Khan and G.I. Evan.Suppression of Myc-induced apoptosis in beta cells exposes multiple oncogenic properties of Myc and triggers carcinogenic progression. *Cell* 2002; 109: 321–334.

[80] Fulda S., W. Wick, M. Weller and K.M. Debatin. Smac agonists sensitize for Apo2L/TRAIL- or anticancer drug-induced apoptosis and induce regression of malignant glioma in vivo. *Nat. Med.* 2002; 8: 808–815.

[81] Fulda S., C. Friesen, M. Los, C. Scaffidi, W. Mier, M. Benedict, G. Nunez, P.H. Krammer, M.E. Peter and K.M. Debatin. Betulinic acid triggers CD95 (APO-1/Fas)-and p53-independent apoptosis via activation of caspases in neuroectodermal tumors. *Cancer Res.* 1997; 57: 4956–4964.

[82] Grotzer M.A., A. Eggert, T.J. Zuzak, A.J. Janss, S. Marwaha, B.R. Wiewrodt, N. Ikegaki, G.M. Brodeur and P.C. Phillips, . Resistance to TRAIL-induced apoptosis in primitive neuroectodermal brain tumor cells correlates with a loss of caspase-8 expression. *Oncogene* 2000; 19:4604–4610.

[83] Hopkins-Donaldson S., A. Ziegler, S. Kurtz, C. Bigosch, D. Kandioler, C. Ludwig, U. Zangemeister-Wittke and R. Stahel. Silencing of death receptor and caspase-8 expression in small cell lung carcinoma cell lines and tumors by DNA methylation. *Cell Death Differ.* 2003; 10:356–364.

[84] Okabe-Kado J. Serum nm23-H1 protein as a prognostic factor in hematological malignancies. *Leuk. Lymphoma* 2002; 43:859–867.

[85] Vogan K., M. Bernstein, J.M. Leclerc, L. Brisson, J. Brossard, G.M. Brodeur, J. Pelletier and P. Gros. Absence of p53 gene mutations in primary neuroblastomas. *Cancer Res*. 1993; 53: 5269–5273.

[86] Moll U.M., M. LaQuaglia, J. Benard and G. Riou. Wild-type p53 protein undergoes cytoplasmic sequestration in undifferentiated neuroblastomas but not in differentiated tumors. *Proc. Natl. Acad. Sci. USA* 1995; 92:4407–4411.

[87] Nikolaev A.Y., M. Li, N. Puskas, J. Qin and W. Gu. Parc: a cytoplasmic anchor for p53. *Cell* 2003; 112:29–40.

[88] Kaghad M., H. Bonnet, A. Yang, L. Creancier, J.C. Biscan, A. Valent, A. Minty, P. Chalon, J.M. Lelias, X. Dumont, P. Ferrara, F. McKeon and D. Caput, . Monoallelically expressed gene related to p53 at 1p36, a region frequently deleted in neuroblastoma and other human cancers. *Cell* 1997; 90:809–819.

[89] Corn P.G., S.J. Kuerbitz, M.M. van Noesel, M. Esteller, N. Compitello, S.B. Baylin and J.G. Herman. Transcriptional silencing of the p73 gene in acute lymphoblastic leukemia and Burkitt's lymphoma is associated with 5' CpG island methylation. *Cancer Res*. 1999; 59:3352–3356.

[90] Casciano I., K. Mazzocco, L. Boni, G. Pagnan, B. Banelli, G. Allemanni, M. Ponzoni, G.P. Tonini and M. Romani. Expression of DeltaNp73 is a molecular marker for adverse outcome in neuroblastoma patients. *Cell Death Differ*. 2002; 9:246–251.

[91] Molenaar J.J., P. van Sluis, K. Boon, R. Versteeg and H.N. Caron. Rearrangements and increased expression of cyclin D1 (CCND1) in neuroblastoma. *Genes Chromosomes Cancer* 2003; 36:242–249.

Index

A

B

D

F

G

H

I

N

O

P

Q

R

S

T

U

V

W

X

Y

Z